- **Fever** over 103° tha
  fever in an infant ur

- **Severe head pain** associated with a stiff neck, drowsiness or pinpoint rash may be a symptom of meningitis, a life-threatening condition. Call your doctor and go to the emergency room.

- **Head injury** if there is loss of consciousness, a decreased level of consciousness or if there is vomiting more than once. If your child falls asleep after the injury, wake her up every thirty minutes to make sure she is still alert.

- **Severe sore throat** that lasts for three days or more accompanied by a fever of more than 103°.

- **Belly pain** that is sudden (acute onset) and is associated with vomiting and no appetite, or if it wakes your child up from sleep.

- **Any bone, joint or muscle pain that persists.** Repeat testing if the pain persists, even if the initial test is negative. Under the age of 2, children express pain through irritability or screaming if you touch or move a part of their bodies that hurts. If this happens, take the baby immediately to the emergency room.

- **Gaping wounds** or **wounds with a flap** need stitching. It is important to go to an emergency room immediately because the wound has to be closed within 6 hours.

- **Burns** that need immediate medical attention:
  — More than two inches square, and/or
  — Blistering, and/or
  — On the face, palm of the hand or genitals

OWN YOUR HEALTH

The Best of Alternative & Conventional Medicine

Your Sick Child

FEVER, ALLERGIES, EAR INFECTIONS,
COLDS AND MORE

JOHN D. MARK, M.D.
STANFORD UNIVERSITY
MEDICAL CENTER

AND ROANNE WEISMAN

ILLUSTRATIONS BY ANN MIYA

Health Communications, Inc.
Deerfield Beach, Florida

www.hcibooks.com

This book is not intended to be a substitute for the advice and/or medical care of the reader's physician. The reader should consult with a physician in all matters related to his or her health.

Library of Congress Cataloging-in-Publication Data
available from the Library of Congress

Publisher: Health Communications, Inc.
         3201 S.W. 15th Street
         Deerfield Beach, FL 33442–8190

Illustrations by Ann Miya, ©2005.
Cover and inside book design by Lawna Patterson Oldfield
Cover photos ©Artville, ©Shutterstock

CONTENTS

PREFACE

To me, "owning my health" means taking as much responsibility as possible for what goes on in my body. It is the opposite of feeling like the helpless victim of pain, disease or disability. It also means working in a collaborative partnership with my doctor to find the best ways to prevent and treat disease from all worlds of medicine: alternative and complementary as well as conventional.

Here is how I learned to "own my health:" In 1995 I woke up from heart valve surgery with the left side of my body paralyzed from a stroke. A tiny piece of tissue had broken away from the valve, traveled through blood vessels and lodged in my brain, blocking the flow of blood with its essential supply of oxygen to the neurons that controlled movement on my left side.

If I had obediently followed the prescribed role of stroke patient in the world of conventional medicine, I would be dependent on adaptive devices and other people for many of the activities of daily life. Instead, I have recovered completely and am back to my life as a medical journalist, wife and mother.

I quickly learned that while the advances of modern medicine can save your life, the conventional medical system—along with the insurers who pay for it—is not set up for true healing. The goal of the system was to get me to a minimal level of functioning, out of the hospital or rehabilitation facility, and back home. What happened after that was up to me.

As a patient, it often feels as if the conventional health care system wants us to accept and "adapt" to our health problems—whether we are recovering from a heart attack or stroke or suffering from chronic illness or pain. We often feel as if we are being treated as collections of body parts to be "fixed" with pills or adaptive devices, rather than as whole people with emotions, relationships, minds and spirits.

By contrast, "integrative medicine," which is the philosophy of this *Own Your Health* book series, encourages people to combine complementary and alternative medicine (often called "CAM") with conventional medicine to find true healing of body, mind and spirit—to achieve wholeness.

As a parent, integrative medicine has particular advantages as you look for ways to provide the best care for your children. As John D. Mark, M.D., notes in his introduction to this book, many parents are dissatisfied with conventional treatments for their children's ear infections, asthma, pain or belly problems and are searching for other options to combine with conventional pediatric treatment.

Going outside of the conventional medical system can be a tough thing to do for those of us who are accustomed to seeing our doctors as omniscient beings who control our health and the health of our families. But when I looked for ways to expand my own healing options, I found many treatments that helped me recover. These included acupuncture and tai chi from the ancient system of Traditional Chinese Medicine; yoga, from the equally ancient Indian Ayurvedic system of medicine; the Alexander Technique—a powerful system of movement education that teaches you to use your body with less effort and reduced pain; craniosacral therapy; and various forms of bodywork and massage. As you will see in this book, these and other healing methods—such as herbal medicine and homeopathy—are also effective for many childhood ailments.

I am grateful that John D. Mark, M.D., of the Stanford University Medical Center, is the coauthor of this book. Not only is he a skilled and caring pediatrician, he is also one of the first two pediatricians in the United States to be awarded a fellowship in pediatric integrative medicine from the National Institutes of Health. He is a specialist in lung diseases of children and has devoted his time to practicing integrative pediatric medicine as well as researching complementary and alternative treatments for many childhood illnesses. Dr. Mark and I also appreciate the expert, compassionate advice of Joy A. Weydert, M.D., FAAP, director of Integrative Pain Management at Children's Mercy Hospital in Kansas City; Lawrence Rosen, M.D., who directs the Maria Fareri Integrative Pediatric Service at Children's Hospital in Westchester County, New York; Russell Greenfield, M.D., Medical Director of Carolinas Integrative Health; and Alexa Fleckenstein, M.D., for her expertise in European Natural Medicine.

Finally, we wish to thank illustrator Ann Miya for helping to bring the concepts of integrative medicine to life. Her drawings, filled with compassion and hope, represent the dreams of all parents for the health, wholeness and happiness of their children.

We hope that this book will help you and your children to "own your health."

—*Roanne Weisman*

INTRODUCTION

When your child is sick it feels as if not much else in life matters. You will do anything to relieve this small person's suffering—whether it means easing pain, restoring comfortable breathing or providing the most nourishing food. But parents often do not know how to make their children feel better, and conventional medical treatments—which may have undesirable side effects—are not always the answer.

I became interested in integrative medicine—the combination of alternative treatments with conventional care—because of such parents. During my years as a general pediatrician, followed by working as the pediatric pulmonary outreach director for Stanford University and the University of California at San Francisco, parents and other practitioners would come to me with questions that I did not have answers for: What are the best alternative therapies for asthma, allergies, ear infections, frequent colds, pain and digestion problems? In many cases, parents were dissatisfied with what the conventional system had to offer and were searching for other ways to help their children. They had heard about alternative treatments from other parents or had done their own research on the Internet.

Although I specialize in lung diseases of children, I also treat other pediatric problems. I soon realized that I needed more tools in my medicine bag and began to learn not only about alternative therapies, but also about the effects of lifestyle on health. This led me to the University of Arizona Program in Integrative Medicine, directed by Dr. Andrew Weil. As part of the Program in Integrative Medicine and the Department of Pediatrics there, I was fortunate to become one of the first two pediatricians in the United States to be awarded a fellowship in pediatric integrative medicine from the National Institutes of Health. I spent two rewarding years conducting research, learning about the different complementary and alternative therapies, and treating children in the clinic and the hospital in an "integrative" manner. After this fellowship, I joined the University of Arizona as assistant professor of clinical pediatrics. Now I am back at Stanford using integrative medicine to treat children, teaching in the medical school and conducting research. While I still treat all childhood illnesses, I am particularly interested in integrating alternative and conventional therapies in the treatment of children with lung problems such as asthma, cystic fibrosis and chronic pneumonia.

In this book, we will help you expand the tools in *your* medicine bag, drawing on the expertise of several physicians who specialize in integrative medicine for children, as well as the findings of research studies to tell you what works and what does not. By using integrative medicine, you not only treat immediate problems, you can also enhance the overall health of your children. We will offer suggestions for creating *balance* in your child's life: Is there anything in your child's diet or environment that may be affecting health? What about stress—in the child as well as the family? What can you as a parent do to prevent *future* health problems for your children? Conventional medicine does not always address these questions well, and that is what we hope to do in this book.

We know that your children mean the world to you, and we want to provide you with the best of *all* worlds of medicine to care for them.

—*John D. Mark, M.D.*

1

THE INTEGRATIVE APPROACH: RESTORE YOUR CHILD'S INNATE HEALING POWER

Our bodies are able to heal themselves, and this is especially true of the growing bodies of our children. We all have innate capacities to restore balance, repair damaged cells and recover from illness. Problems arise when these natural healing abilities are blocked, either by stress, poor diet or a lifestyle that demands too much of us. Conventional medicine is good at treating the symptoms of illness but is less effective at helping to stimulate our own natural healing abilities.

Integrative medicine, on the other hand, recognizes that we are more than the cells, molecules and atoms that make up our bodies. We all have something else—something that won't show up on an x-ray or CT scan. We can call this our life force, soul, spirit, energy or many other names. But whatever we call it, it is this intangible "energy" that gives us the power to recover and repair our bodies from the stress, bacteria, viruses, pollution, injuries and other onslaughts that most of us deal with every day. The suggestions in this book are designed to help you work with your health care provider to give your children the resilience they need to live, grow and flourish at home and at school.

To make the book easy to navigate, we have divided up the chapters according to health problems as they appear in different areas of the body. There are also chapters discussing overall problems, such as pain, stress and insomnia. We have included "A Closer Look" sections to describe some alternative therapies that merit attention and "What's the Evidence?" sections to let you know about therapies that research has found to be effective.

A Guide to the Integrative Approach: When to Question Your Pediatrician

Many parents are faced with medical advice from their pediatricians that they might want to question, but have a hard time doing so. I encourage you to ask questions about the wisdom of conventional treatments and the value of alternative methods. If you feel your pediatrician might not respond well to being questioned, you might phrase it this way: "I've heard that antibiotics, especially for first-time ear infections, may not be the best treatment, and that homeopathy is effective and safe. What do you think about that?" or "I've heard that biofeedback for migraines and asthma (or osteopathy for digestive problems) may be treatment options to consider. What's your opinion?"

You might also want to check, in a nonthreatening way, to make sure your pediatrician is keeping up with the latest literature on both conventional and integrative medicine. ("Have you heard about the latest recommendations about keeping to a normal diet for diarrhea? Aren't they interesting?") Trust your instincts about what is best. No one knows your child better than you!

Medical Recommendations to Be Wary Of

Here are some "red flags" that should encourage you to seek out other opinions and more information:

- *Automatic prescription of antibiotics, especially strong ones.* For first-time ear infections, the integrative approach is "watchful waiting," along with the nonmedication practices described in Chapter 3, "Earaches and Ear Infections." If you and your pediatrician agree to use an antibiotic for recurrent ear infections, amoxicillin is still the antibiotic of choice. Stronger antibiotics, such as Ciprofloxacin, should never be given to children under fifteen without a very good reason.
- *Ear tubes.* These should be used as a last resort, after all conventional and alternative methods have failed for recurrent or persistent ear infections with documented hearing loss.
- *Food restrictions for diarrhea.* The latest research supports the idea of giving children a regular diet, even through diarrheal illness. The older approach of clear liquids and the "BRAT" (banana, rice, applesauce, toast) diet is found to be less desirable and may actually prolong the illness.
- *Cow's milk, cheese and butter.* As you will see in Chapters 2 and 3, cow's milk and other dairy products may exacerbate inflammation in the airways and other parts of the body. My

approach, and that of most other integrative physicians, is to limit or eliminate cow's milk, cheese and butter from the diets of children with chronic medical problems, especially because so many children (and adults) have trouble digesting it (lactose intolerance). There are other sources of calcium, vitamins and protein, despite what the dairy industry would have us believe. These include green, leafy vegetables; nuts; calcium-fortified juices and cereals; legumes and beans.

- *Immediate treatment of low-grade fever.* Fever is the body's way of slowing and even killing viruses and bacteria, and I would not rush to acetaminophen or ibuprofen right away. There are many other ways to make a child comfortable described in Chapter 6, "Colds and Fever." Of course, call your doctor if your child has a persistent high fever (over 103 degrees) or for any fever in an infant under two months.

Family Health Care with Integrative Medicine: A Positive Example

Maureen and Walter live in a large Victorian house that is filled with books on homeopathy and

Traditional Chinese Medicine. "For the past ten years we have used the best family medicine from both the conventional and alternative worlds," says Maureen. This health strategy has helped the family cope not only with serious problems—such as the failure to thrive of their youngest child, Emmett, when he was an infant—but also with the everyday problems of childhood illnesses for all three children.

It was Maureen's experiences with Emmett, when he was diagnosed as "failing to thrive," that led her to integrative medicine. After fourteen months of almost constant vomiting, Emmett was finally diagnosed (after lengthy testing and food analyses) with an inability to digest fruit sugars. He was treated in a collaboration between his conventional doctors and a homeopathic physician whom Maureen finally consulted. "We always made sure that every health professional, whether conventional or alternative, knew everything that we were doing with Emmett," says Maureen. Today Emmett is a happy, curious high-school student with a great sense of humor. He is doing well in school and enjoys acting, singing and soccer. "He understands very well the connection between fruit products and his digestion and has learned to read labels and ask questions before he eats anything that might contain fruit by-products," says Maureen.

Emmett's failure-to-thrive condition left him with a somewhat compromised immune system, according to Maureen. "Although he is healthy now, he has less stamina than other kids, and is more prone to colds and bronchitis," she says. "When he was nine, he had viral meningitis and mononucleosis. We found that combining alternative and complementary treatments with his conventional health care has helped him overcome illnesses fairly quickly." Looking back on their experiences with Emmett, Maureen comments, "His digestion problem took fourteen months to diagnose and showed us both the strengths and weaknesses of allopathic [conventional] medicine. We feel that Emmett would not be who he is today without the interventions of conventional medical science *together with* homeopathy, acupuncture and other complementary treatments."

Maureen also found that a Japanese style of acupuncture that includes magnet therapy is often helpful when the children feel run down. "I learned to put the magnets on them at home, and it seems to help when they think they are coming down with something. Sometimes we can ward it off," she says. "Another preventive treatment is a constitutional remedy that our homeopathic physician has developed specifically for Emmett's personal characteristics. He takes this a few times a year." Maureen also keeps a homeopathic remedy kit at home. "There are remedies for all kinds of acute ailments, including colds, coughs, flu, stomach problems and ear infections, and I have learned so much about using them through reading and consulting with our homeopathic physician, who is also our pediatrician and primary care family practitioner," she says. "We have all benefited."

Maureen used an additional complementary therapy for her daughter. "When Emileigh was in kindergarten, she fell and hit her head on a rock," says Maureen. "There was no concussion, but she needed stitches. We put ice on it and didn't think much more about it. But she soon began having headaches and reading problems, so we had her vision tested and found out that she needed glasses." Emileigh wore the glasses until second grade, but then Maureen decided once more to look beyond conventional medical treatment.

"The glasses did not seem to be alleviating all of her headaches and reading complaints, so I took her to a craniosacral practitioner," says Maureen. (See "A Closer Look at Osteopathy and Craniosacral Therapy.") "Cradling Emileigh's head, the practitioner gently made tiny adjustments in the connections, called 'sutures,' that join the bones of the skull, particularly in the area that affects vision. We think that the fall knocked something out of alignment. After two sessions, her headaches were gone; and at her next vision checkup she no longer needed glasses." Emileigh, now an athletic college freshman, has not worn glasses since.

2

ASTHMA, SINUS PROBLEMS, ALLERGIES, CHRONIC BRONCHITIS AND OTHER RESPIRATORY PROBLEMS

A four-year-old girl imagines a tightly closed rosebud opening its petals to become a beautiful flower. A twelve-year-old boy sees a complex arrangement of pipes with valves turned to the "on" position. A teenager visualizes a narrow stream that becomes a cascading mountain waterfall. As they close their eyes and think of these images, the children feel their airways open and they can breathe more freely. All three have asthma, a chronic inflammation of the lungs that restricts breathing, and all of them have learned "guided imagery" techniques that help open their airways, often without the use of asthma drugs.

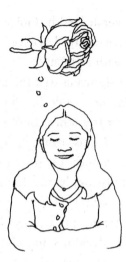

Asthma is the leading cause of chronic illness in children and teens. The number of children with asthma in the United States has more than doubled in the past fifteen years. For preschool and school-age children, asthma has reached epidemic proportions.[1] Conventional treatment of asthma includes medications such as inhaled steroids, which may have side effects. Many health care practitioners treat only the symptoms of a child with asthma instead of the underlying condition causing the symptoms. Integrative physicians use safe, effective alternative therapies in addition to conventional medications to minimize side effects and improve overall health. Guided imagery and visualization have emerged as excellent options for many children with asthma.

Research has shown us that the mind can influence the body, not only in the treatment of asthma, but for many other childhood illnesses as well. If you doubt this, think of squeezing a tart lemon into your mouth. Do you begin to salivate? Guided imagery is simply a technique of creating images and thoughts in your mind that are directed to particular areas of your body. I have seen patients, both adults and children, use this technique to slow down a too-rapid heartbeat, increase blood flow to icy hands, or relax the stomach and internal organs to ease pain and improve digestion.

With training, the mind can actually change the immunological response to disease. For example, we can teach children with asthma to use visualization and the power of the mind to open airways, reducing both mucous and inflammation in the lungs. Young kids are great at relaxing—they daydream naturally and their imaginations are so active. Children between six and twelve have some of the most creative visualizations of any age group.

TEACHING GUIDED IMAGERY AND VISUALIZATION TO CHILDREN

Advocates of guided imagery contend that the imagination is a potent healer, that we can use images in our minds to make changes in our bodies, and there is data to back this up. Images and other senses are thought to be a way for the brain to communicate with the organs of the body. In fact, imagery has been referred to as the "language" that the mind uses to communicate with the body. "We can't eliminate all the stress in our children's lives, but we can give them tools such as guided imagery, visualization and biofeedback to help them manage that stress," says Lawrence Rosen, M.D., director of the Integrative Pediatric Service at Maria Fareri Children's Hospital in Westchester County, New York. "We can use these tools to help children feel more in control of their situations, whether they are having trouble sleeping, experiencing performance or test anxiety, or having chronic pain or digestive problems. For example, the child can use breathing and relaxation techniques and then visualize a place where she feels calm, safe and relaxed." Dr. Rosen suggests that parents use videos or professional training to learn how to teach these skills to children. (See "Resources" at the end of this book as well as the sidebar "Teach Your Child to Relax" in Chapter 8.)

Asthma—An Integrative Approach

The primary conventional treatment for persistent asthma is the use of steroids through an inhaler. My goal with children is to use the conventional treatment initially, to establish control of their asthma, but then to taper off and even discontinue these medicines as soon as possible. We do this by finding out which alternative approaches both the child and the family can accept. This is what integrative medicine is all about.

One of my patients was a five-year-old girl who was coughing almost all night long and whenever she tried to exercise. She also had frequent colds and bronchitis. She was irritable and tired during the day because of her sleep interruptions, and she was often too sick to participate in family activities. The parents, however, did not want to accept the diagnosis of asthma, primarily because they did not like the idea of their child inhaling steroids. I began by working with the family to help them see the need for medication to give her relief at night and to control the chronic inflammation. They were able to accept this after they understood it would not be permanent. They also saw that it helped their daughter sleep.

While she was taking the medication, I also worked with her and her parents to adjust her diet, talked about lifestyle and began to teach her guided imagery/visualization techniques. After just a few weeks on the medication, this child was able to control her asthma symptoms on her own, through a combination of changes in what she ate, guided imagery and the addition of dietary supplements. Eventually, she no longer needed medication. As I mentioned earlier, even very young children can learn guided imagery, and there are practitioners who can help you teach them. (See "Resources" at the end of this book.)

Treating Asthma, Chronic Bronchitis and Other Upper Respiratory Problems

Do not treat your child alone, with these or any other suggestions. Always consult with your pediatrician. Use conventional medication when recommended by your doctor, but try to wean the child off it with alternative therapies, including:

- *Visualization and guided imagery* (as described earlier in this chapter).
- *Dietary changes*. Polyunsaturated and hydrogenated fats, which are in almost every

cookie, snack and cracker, increase the inflammatory response in the body. Because asthma and other upper respiratory problems are caused by inflammation in the lungs, the fewer of such foods your child eats, the better. Check food labels carefully, and try to encourage your child to eat more fresh fruits and vegetables and stay away from processed foods. The general rule is: The fresher the better!

- *Exercise.* Encourage swimming, biking, rollerskating, yoga or martial arts. Aerobic exercise helps with breathing and reducing the frequency and duration of colds. Martial arts and yoga are particularly beneficial for children with asthma because they teach *control* of the breath.

Some people's asthma may be made worse with exercise, especially if their asthma is not under control or they are exposed to adverse conditions such as cold, dry air; wind; or particulates (like a dust storm or during an ozone warning). There is also a portion of the population with exercise-induced asthma (including famous Olympic athletes Nancy Hogshead and Jim Ryan). However, children and adults who have asthma that is stable and under control can often benefit from exercise. It helps them use their lungs to full capacity and develop stamina and respiratory muscle strength, and often will help decrease the amount of medication needed. Activities such as swimming and other sports that occur in a more "humid" environment (cold, dry air can exacerbate asthma) are popular; however, studies show that any type of exercise is good for stable asthma. People with exercise-induced asthma can premedicate with certain inhalers (albuterol, salmeterol, cromolyn sodium) to "block" the symptoms. Slow warm-ups can also lessen exercise symptoms.

- *Dietary supplements*. For children **over the age of five**, use dietary supplements, including a good multivitamin with vitamins C, A and E as well as selenium. There has been some research showing that B-complex vitamins and antioxidants help lung function.[2] There is also evidence that fish oils, especially omega-3 fatty acids, are helpful, so encourage your child to eat more salmon, sardines, mackerel and herring.

- *Manual therapy*. Osteopathy,[3] massage therapy[4] and other manual therapy techniques have been shown to improve symptoms of asthma and increase lung function in both children and adults. (See "A Closer Look" sections for a description of these and other alternative treatments.)

Treating Sinus Problems and Allergies

The asthma remedies described above can also be helpful for allergy and sinus symptoms. Additional suggestions:

- *Analyze environmental history* to determine if the symptoms may be coming from pets, house dust mites (found in bedding, carpets and upholstery) or pollen.
- *Investigate possible food allergies.* Many children with chronic respiratory problems do better if they cut out milk, cheese, ice cream, butter and other dairy products. Other possible culprits are food dyes from processed foods. Try eliminating dairy and as many processed foods as possible for at least two weeks to see if there is any change in symptoms. Sometimes food cravings can be a clue to an allergy. One conventional allergist

recommends eliminating for two weeks any food that the child craves to see if it makes a difference in symptoms.

- *Acupuncture* (if children will tolerate it) helps alleviate asthma as well as allergy symptoms in some children.[5]
- *Sinus irrigation.* (See sidebar "Sinus Irrigation for Ear, Throat and Upper Respiratory Infections" in Chapter 3.)

WHAT'S THE EVIDENCE?

Complementary Therapies for Asthma, Allergies and Upper Respiratory Infections

While the following studies relate to asthma, they are also applicable to allergies and upper respiratory infections.

Hands-On Therapy Works for Children (and Adults)

When parents, after instruction, spent twenty minutes a night giving massage therapy to their children, the children showed improved lung function, decreased need for medication and reduced asthma symptoms.[6] Osteopathic manipulation in an emergency room improved lung function and breathing in adults.[7]

The Mind-Body Connection

Yoga,[8] acupuncture[9] and relaxation techniques, including guided imagery and self-hypnosis,[10] were also found to be helpful for symptom relief.

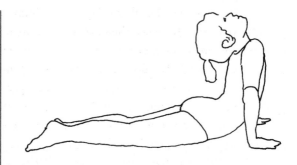

Guided Imagery and Visualization

Studies have shown that guided imagery, also referred to as self-hypnosis, is most successful when used in conjunction with relaxation techniques such as meditation and yoga.[11] From this relaxed state patients can create images that include airways opening up, pain receding or a heart beating in a normal rhythm. Often, these images have physiological impact.

Several randomized, controlled studies indicate that these techniques are beneficial for children and adults with asthma. However, these studies should be viewed with caution. With a few exceptions, there has been little research on guided imagery and visualization for childhood asthma focusing on objective pulmonary (lung) function measurements.

One study did find that relaxation training in children not only helped their asthma, as measured by pulmonary function tests, medication use and symptoms, but also decreased airway inflammation.[12] The use of storytelling, imagery and relaxation in a family asthma education program resulted in improvements in medication use, asthma scores and symptoms in preschool children.[13] And a study of adults found that treatment with a "hypnotic technique" resulted in improvements for adults with moderate asthma.[14]

A CLOSER LOOK

Osteopathy and Craniosacral Therapy: Movement Is All

"Osteopaths focus on the structure of the body and how it functions," explains Rachel Brooks, M.D. "The goal is to restore the free, natural flow of movement at all levels, whether in the bones and joints, muscles and ligaments, the organs within their sheaths of connective tissue, or the flow of blood, lymph fluid or the cerebrospinal fluid that bathes and cushions the spinal cord and nerves throughout the body." Dr. Brooks lives in Portland, Oregon, and is a graduate of the University of

Michigan Medical School "Though an M.D. by training, I've devoted my whole professional life to osteopathy," she says.

Dr. Andrew Taylor Still, a physician who served in the Union Army, founded osteopathy in the late 1800s. "After his wife and children died in an epidemic of spinal meningitis, Dr. Still became disillusioned with the tools of allopathic medicine," says Dr. Brooks. "He developed osteopathy as a hands-on way to treat people that built on what he believed to be the body's own inherent capacity to heal." Dr. Still developed a method of using the hands to affect the structure of the body to encourage and restore the free and natural flow of movement on every level. Some of the key principles of osteopathy are:

1. The body is a unit; the person is a unit of body, mind and spirit.
2. The body is capable of self-regulation, self-healing and health maintenance.
3. The structure and function of the whole body are related.

There are a number of manipulative approaches in osteopathy. Dr. Brooks practices a type called "cranial osteopathy," an extremely gentle practice that she uses to treat problems related to injury and illness. She can use the method to treat ear infections in children, pain resulting from muscle strain or trauma, infections and menstrual problems.

Our bodies are never still, says Dr. Brooks. In addition to the beating of our hearts and the breath that flows in and out of our lungs, there is a constant pulse of movement throughout our organs and tissues. "Cranial osteopaths work from the principle that this constant, natural 'pulsing' within the body is how the body maintains itself in a state of health," she says, explaining that this pulsing has been linked to the slow, rhythmic movement of the cerebrospinal fluid originally described by osteopathic physician William Garner Sutherland in the 1930s. "By finding out where this rhythm is blocked, whether it is caused by injury or illness, and then helping the body to release that blockage, we can reduce pain and restore health," says Dr. Brooks. "For example, promoting a greater flow of lymph fluid, which helps to clear infection, allows the body to work more efficiently to recover from pneumonia and other infectious diseases."

Osteopathy for Ear Infections

Dr. Brooks explains how cranial osteopathy works, using childhood ear infections as an example. "Many people think of the head as a solid 'bowling ball' type of structure, but that is not the case," she says. "The bones of a newborn's skull are moveable and then become connected by seams called 'sutures' as the child grows. The skull solidifies, but even in the adult it always retains a resilience in the suture connections. I could train you to place your hands on someone's head and feel the slight, rhythmic, rocking movement that is normally present." The ear, Dr. Brooks explains, is located in a chamber inside the temporal bone of the skull, on either side of the head. "If something, either a birth trauma or an injury, jams the temporal bone, limiting its natural rocking motion, the fluids that flow inside the ear cannot drain normally," she says. "And if fluid is relatively still and stagnant, it is more prone to infection."

Dr. Brooks explains that in every case she first examines the whole body to find out where the restrictions are, even if they are not located near the area of the symptoms. "Often, restrictions elsewhere in the body can have important effects on the area where the symptoms are," she explains. To treat the temporal bone, Dr. Brooks holds the head while the patient is lying on a table. Following the body's own rhythm, she uses gentle, barely perceptible motions to encourage the free movement of the temporal bones. "I do not apply a significant force from the outside," she says. "I use my hands and my own intention to help the body find a state of balance and support while allowing the tissues to release. I have found colicky, irritable babies respond well to this treatment, as well as adults with head or neck injuries and pain."

Over the years since Dr. Still created the practice of osteopathy, it has entered into the field of mainstream medicine. Doctors of osteopathy (D.O.) are certified to practice all medical specialties, including surgery. However, they add a more holistic approach through their special training in osteopathic manipulation.

Cranial Osteopathy and Craniosacral Therapy for Children

While general osteopathy and cranial osteopathy are performed by doctors of osteopathy, a similar treatment, called "craniosacral therapy," can be performed by other practitioners, such as chiropractors, massage therapists, nurses and physical therapists. Craniosacral therapy grew out of the system of osteopathy and treats the central nervous system and its relationship to the spinal cord in a similar way. The craniosacral "rhythm" within the body comes from the regular pulsing of the liquid— called "cerebrospinal fluid"—that bathes, nourishes and protects the spinal cord. It is through the regular pulses of the cerebrospinal fluid that the brain transmits nerve signals to keep the body alive and functioning.

Russell Greenfield, M.D., a former emergency room physician who is medical director of Carolinas Integrative Health in Charlotte, North Carolina, often refers children for cranial osteopathy. "I prefer cranial osteopathy, provided by an osteopath, as part of an overall medical treatment," says Dr. Greenfield. "When treating an adult or a child, you want to make sure that the whole body is being evaluated for imbalances, including the skull, facial bones, sacrum, limbs, ribs, pelvis, muscles and organs. I feel that osteopaths are best equipped to perform this kind of evaluation." Dr. Greenfield recommends cranial osteopathy for the following childhood problems in select instances:

- Recurrent ear infections
- Mild seizure disorders (only in rare cases)
- Temporomandibular joint (TMJ) pain
- Autism
- Attention deficit hyperactivity disorder (ADHD)
- Learning disability
- Birth trauma
- Developmental disorders
- Headaches, including migraines

- Asthma
- Recurrent sinusitis

In my own practice, I have seen benefits to children both from cranial osteopathy performed by doctors of osteopathy, as well as craniosacral therapy performed by other well-trained practitioners. As Dr. Greenfield points out, the most important component in effective treatment is that the practitioner takes into account the condition of the entire body, and that neither of these techniques replaces necessary conventional treatment.

While there is a need for better research on the effectiveness of both cranial osteopathy and craniosacral therapy, experience suggests that both of these treatments, performed by skilled, experienced practitioners, may be reasonable options for parents to consider in conditions for which conventional medicine has little to offer. "We don't understand everything there is to know about health and healing," says Dr. Greenfield about osteopathy. "But there is plausibility behind the theories of osteopathy and safety associated with the interventions when applied by well-trained practitioners. Parents can reasonably consider osteopathic manipulation as a treatment for their children."

WHAT'S THE EVIDENCE?

Osteopathy and Craniosacral Therapy

Research on osteopathy is not plentiful and needs to be broadened, but several studies show a benefit for children with asthma, recurrent ear infections,[15] developmental delays[16] and attention-deficit disorders.[17] In addition, studies indicate that it is effective for musculoskeletal pain,[18] especially for post-operative recovery and lower back pain, although one study found no significant difference between osteopathic treatment and standard medical care.[19]

Craniosacral Therapy

No controlled trials of craniosacral therapy seem to exist, according to one author, Dr. Edzard Ernst, who surveyed the literature, pointing out that Dr. Upledger himself, who developed the technique, does not cite them in his own writing. "Even though small movements between cranial bones are possible, there is no good evidence to suggest that restrictions of these movements have any health related relevance," writes Dr. Ernst.[20]

However, practitioners, patients and parents

claim that the technique is beneficial for problems such as birth trauma, chronic pain, cerebral dysfunction, cerebral palsy, colic, depression, dyslexia, ear infections, headaches, learning disabilities, Ménière's disease, musculoskeletal problems, migraine, sinusitis and stroke. Young children are believed to respond particularly well.

3

EARACHES

AND

EAR INFECTIONS

As almost any parent of young children knows, ear infections can occur with depressing regularity. They are common in young children because the mechanism that drains fluid from the middle ear is not yet well developed, making this a fertile breeding ground for bacteria and viruses to accumulate and cause infection, fluid buildup and pain.

To reduce the risk of ear infections and many other health problems, breast-feeding is strongly encouraged for the first six months of life (at least) and secondhand smoke should be eliminated from the child's environment.

The conventional treatment for childhood ear infections is usually a course of antibiotics, but concern is rising that overuse of antibiotics is leading to ever more powerful drug-resistant bacteria. As I noted in an earlier chapter, you should be wary of precipitous use of strong antibiotics. Amoxicillin is still the antibiotic of choice for ear infections. Stronger antibiotics, such as Ciprofloxacin, should never be given to children under fifteen without a very good reason. You should also question carefully a recommendation for ear tubes, especially in young children. Ear tubes should be used as a last resort, after all conventional and alternative methods have failed, for recurrent or persistent ear infections with documented hearing loss.

Many pediatricians, myself included, are now adopting a "watchful-waiting" approach, holding off on the antibiotics and using alternative methods, including:

- *Dietary changes*. Children who are prone to ear infections should never be fed by "bottle propping." A period of avoiding cow's milk and dairy products may decrease the incidence of persistent or recurrent ear infections. However, such products as yogurt, due to their probiotics, may actually help prevent ear infections. If your child has an ear infection, give plenty of warm fluids, including soups and herbal teas, fresh vegetables, and fresh fruit.

- *Aromatherapy.* Use a warm compress laced with essential oils of lavender or chamomile to lessen pain while drawing out the infection by enhancing inner ear function. You can also gently massage around the outer ear with 1-2 drops essential oils diluted in 1 tsp. of vegetable oil. You can find bottles of essential oils at health food stores. Test this first on a small area of skin for one hour to check for any sensitivity before applying extensively. **Never give essential oils internally or apply undiluted directly to the skin.**

- *Hydrotherapy.* Some professionals recommend alternating hot and cold compresses to increase circulation, decrease pressure in the ear area and increase the absorption of inflammatory deposits in the ear. **With any use of compresses, carefully test the temperature on your own skin before applying it to your child, to avoid scalding.**

- *Cranial osteopathy, including craniosacral therapy.* These are methods of manual therapy involving massage, subtle mobilization of the skull bones and gentle spinal manipulation. (See "A Closer Look at Osteopathy and Craniosacral Therapy.") For ear infections, the theory is that an inner ear structure or function may not be working optimally because it is blocked. If a baby was stuck in the birth canal, for example, the function of his or her ear canals may be affected by minute structural changes of the skull from the delivery process, making the child more prone to ear infections. Gentle osteopathic therapies, especially craniosacral manipulation, may restore the proper structure and subsequent normal function.

- *Acupuncture/acupressure.* (See "A Closer Look at Acupuncture and Traditional Chinese Medicine.")

The following homeopathic and herbal remedies for ear infections are recommended by Joy A. Weydert, M.D., FAAP, director, Integrative Pain Management, Children's Mercy Hospital, Kansas City, Missouri. **Note that homeopathic remedies are different from herbs and should be prescribed by a homeopathic physician.**

- *Homeopathic remedies.* Chamomilla, bella-donna, pulsatilla, Kali muraticum, aconite—used alone or in combination may reduce pain associated with ear infections. **Use only in consultation with your pediatrician or a homeopathic physician.**
- *Chamomile.* This herb is calming and anti-spasmodic. Use as a tea or extract three to four times a day orally following package dosing instructions.
- *Echinacea.* This herb boosts the immune system to fight infection. You can use it as a tea, extract or capsule every few hours at the onset of illness, then four times a day until symptoms clear.
- *Warm herbal oils instilled in the ear with an eye-dropper for pain relief.* Use St. John's wort, mullein, garlic, calendula (alone or in combination) infused in olive oil. Ready-made herbal oils can be found in health food stores. **Do not use if child has ear tubes, has ear drainage, or is to be examined by a physician. This will block viewing of the eardrum.**

SINUS IRRIGATION FOR EAR, THROAT AND UPPER RESPIRATORY INFECTIONS

Sinus irrigation, also known as sinus wash or lavage, is a simple procedure that can increase drainage of the sinuses. For children with seasonal allergies, sinus irrigation can remove pollen from the nose. It can also help with upper respiratory infections and colds and be useful for certain types of asthma that include upper respiratory symptoms. It has been recommended by physicians for decades, and its use dates further back in traditional Eastern practices.

The technique uses an "isotonic saline solution," which has a similar salt concentration to body fluids. To make the solution, you will need the following ingredients:

- 1 teaspoon salt—kosher, canning, pickling, or sea salt is preferable to table salt
- 16 ounces water (0.47 liter or 1 U.S. pint), at room temperature
- 1 teaspoon baking soda

Instructions:

1. Mix the ingredients in a clean container with a tight cover. This recipe can be halved and can be used for seven days. Do not store for longer than seven days.

2. Insert solution into a clean rubber-topped dropper. If unavailable, an ear syringe, neti pot (a teapot for the nose) or clean hand can be used. You can also wash a dropper from an empty tincture bottle

3. Place some solution in the upper nostril. Plug that nostril and tilt the head slightly to the opposite side so the fluid runs out the other nostril. Place some more fluid in the nostril and tilt the head slightly backward and to the same side to reach the sinuses. Repeat this procedure with the other nostril. Wash the dropper with hot water each time before dipping it into the saline solution to prevent contamination.

4. Gargle with the same solution, letting it wash the back of your throat.

5. Blow your nose gently.

Precautions and Risks: No swallowing the salty liquid! Over-irrigation can compromise the ability of the sinuses to fight bacteria. Children with acute sinusitis should not be given this procedure, because it can facilitate the spread of bacteria and cause more serious infection. If your child has a deficient immune system, consult your pediatrician before trying this procedure.

A CLOSER LOOK

Homeopathy: Like Cures Like

The practice of homeopathy continues to engender controversy. It is worth taking a closer look at because many people, myself included, recommend it as a gentle, effective, noninvasive way to treat many childhood illnesses. There is research to support this view, but there are also many scientists and physicians who criticize the research, saying it is invalid. This section is meant to give you information about the pros and cons of this therapy and to encourage you, if you are interested, to explore further with your pediatrician and a homeopathic physician like Jennifer Jacobs.

Twenty-five years ago, family practice physician Jennifer Jacobs, M.D., MPH, was looking for "a kinder, gentler way to treat people." She found what she was looking for in homeopathy, a medical system created two hundred years ago by German physician Dr. Samuel Hahnemann, who was himself on a similar quest. "Hahnemann was disillusioned by the harmful medical practices of his day and set out to find a gentler approach," explains Dr. Kenneth R. Pelletier in his comprehensive survey of complementary and alternative medicine.[21]

"Homeopathy is a wonderful way to treat children because it is gentle, nontoxic and effective," says Dr. Jacobs. The treatment is based on the principle that "like cures like." The theory is that tiny amounts of a substance that might cause disease symptoms in healthy people, when given in a highly diluted form to sick people, can stimulate their bodies' natural healing ability to fight the disease. Dr. Jacobs uses an onion to illustrate her point. "When we peel onions we get watery eyes, a runny nose and sometimes a hoarse cough, even though we are not sick. If we take a homeopathic remedy called *Allium cepa*, which is made from the red onion, and give it in a highly diluted form to someone who has these cold symptoms, it helps to stimulate the body to fight the symptoms."

How does homeopathy work? The system is often explained through the concept of a "vital force," which has been called "the organizing, animating principle that maintains health in a living system. . . . A properly selected homeopathic remedy is believed to provoke the vital force so that the body's own healing power can produce the cure."[22] When this energy flow is blocked or obstructed, disease results.

"Many parents do not want to keep giving their children antibiotics for ear infections," says Dr. Jacobs. "And in fact, an antibiotic crisis is underway in this country. Doctors are prescribing antibiotics for viral illnesses, colds and flu, when they are neither necessary nor appropriate. This is creating antibiotic-resistant bacteria, so that when we really do need these medicines—for such diseases as pneumonia, kidney infection or meningitis—they may not work."

Homeopathy is a possible solution to antibiotics, says Dr. Jacobs. "In twenty-five years of treating children with ear infections, I have prescribed antibiotics only once," she says. "With antibiotics, ear infections keep coming back, and they are harder and harder to get rid of. I often see children who are caught in this 'antibiotic treadmill.' I use homeopathic remedies to break the cycle, and they respond beautifully. The body's immune system is strengthened, and there are fewer infections."

Dr. Jacobs's pilot study of ear infections, published in 2001, found that homeopathic remedies for ear infections produced significant decreases in overall symptoms, including pain and fever in the first twenty-four hours when compared to a placebo. In his own review of other research studies, Dr. Pelletier cites evidence that supports the effectiveness of homeopathy for some conditions. "Homeopathy has always been considered particularly helpful for children," he writes. "It is reported to resolve, gently and effectively, such problems as teething pain, hyperactivity, emotional problems, and even learning disabilities. . . . Many parents prefer homeopathy, since pharmaceutical drugs can have unpredictable and long-lasting, even toxic effects on children."[23]

When Dr. Jacobs first meets a new patient or family, she spends more than an hour in an initial interview and examination. "I take the health history, including details about current symptoms and past illnesses," she says. "I also ask about food cravings, sleep patterns, lifestyle, stress, the family situation and such personal details as whether they get cold or warm easily." Dr. Jacobs then uses this information to perform a detailed analysis of the patient's health and to select which homeopathic remedies would be best. "There are thousands of homeopathic remedies," she says. "We have three thousand in our clinic alone, but we commonly use about one hundred. [For examples of specific homeopathic remedies for certain conditions, see chapters on those conditions in this book.] Each remedy is carefully selected to meet the particular constellation of symptoms of each patient." Jacobs stresses that homeopathy does not try to suppress symptoms in the way that antihistamines, for example, suppress cold or allergy symptoms. "These symptoms, whether they are sneezing, a runny nose or diarrhea, are the body's way of trying to heal itself," she explains. "The cold symptoms are a method for expelling bacteria and viruses out of the body. Through diarrhea, the body may be trying to quickly get rid of food-borne bacteria that are damaging the intestinal tract. Fever is a way for the body to kill disease-causing bacteria or viruses with high temperatures."

Homeopathy supports the body's natural ability to heal itself by *building up* the immune response, rather than trying to stop it. "We do this by trying to enhance the response that the body is already making, using the symptoms as a guide to the correct homeopathic remedy," Dr. Jacobs says. "Chronic diarrhea, for example, may be related to stress as well as physical or emotional upset in a person's life. We need to understand its cause in order to match the person with the best remedies." She says that homeopathy can be effective in the treatment of autoimmune diseases as well. "We have had good results with eczema, fibromyalgia, chronic fatigue and irritable bowel. We have even helped people with multiple sclerosis remain stable for five or six years, although we obviously can't reverse the course of the disease, especially if there has been damage to the tissues." Dr. Jacobs also describes good results for the use of homeopathy in the treatment of children with sleep disorders and emotional problems and is studying the use of homeopathy in the treatment of attention deficit hyperactivity disorder.

Homeopathy does not truly fall into the category of "complementary medicine," points out Dr. Jacobs, because it is best used as a stand-alone system. "The system was designed as an alternative to conventional medicine," she says. "Some conventional medical treatments may interfere with the homeopathic remedies. I usually ask my patients to give homeopathy six months to see if it works, and during that time not to add *any new* medicines or treatments to what they are already doing, so we can see clearly what the homeopathy is doing. If they are taking medicines that are optional, they may want to give them up during that time." Of course, all drug decisions should also be made in consultation with your pediatrician.

When to Use Homeopathy at Home; When to Go to the Doctor

Doctors divide illness, particularly childhood illnesses, into two categories: acute and chronic. With a homeopathic remedy kit at home and proper instruction about its use, you can treat many acute childhood illnesses yourself. These include colds, flu, earaches, diarrhea, teething, colic, chicken pox, croup and conjunctivitis. Chronic problems are more difficult to diagnose and treat at home, and for these—which include chronic skin problems, headaches, gastrointestinal problems, recurrent ear infections and behavior problems— you should consult a homeopathic doctor for your child.

WHAT'S THE EVIDENCE?

Homeopathy:
Research and Controversy

Despite the research findings that point to its effectiveness for various medical problems, scientists and conventional medical professionals often criticize homeopathy, and the practice is still extremely controversial. "The idea that microscopic amounts of medicine can cure disease goes against the principles of physics and modern medicine," says one researcher who is opposed to homeopathy. But other researchers argue that studies using principles of quantum physics and electromagnetic energy identified "measurable and unique electromagnetic signals emitted by homeopathic remedies. The signals produced specific dominant frequencies for each homeopathic substance tested."[24] This was found to be true even in remedies where no molecule of the original substance remained. Several studies supporting this view are reviewed by Linda W. Freeman, Ph.D., in her 2001 article, "Homeopathy—A Scientific Enigma."[25] Supporters of homeopathy also point out that the principle of "like cures like" is the basis for the development of vaccines and allergy desensitization treatments. Dr. Pelletier takes some issue with this notion. "This analogy, though, is not really accurate, since the substances used in immunization and desensitization are identical or similar to the disease-causing agents, whereas homeopathic remedies are usually substances different from those that cause disease."[26]

Even as the controversy continues, scientific evidence in support of homeopathy appears to be growing. Dr. Freeman cites research reporting that homeopathy is effective for digestive disorders, chronic fatigue, treatment for allergies, otitis media (acute or chronic ear infections), immune dysfunction, colic in babies, short-term acute illnesses, such as influenza, and chronic pain syndromes, such as migraine.

Two reviews of homeopathic research trials showed the effectiveness of homeopathy. One, published in 1991 in the *British Medical Journal*, found that out of 107 controlled clinical trials of homeopathy, 81 showed that homeopathic medicines had some positive results, and 24 showed no positive effects. (Two were inconclusive.) Conditions that benefited from homeopathy included vascular disease, respiratory infections, hay fever, faster return of bowel function following abdominal surgery, rheumatological disorders, pain or trauma, and mental or psychological problems. However, the authors caution that publication bias (due to the controversy surrounding homeopathy) and poor methodology may have complicated the results of the review. [27]

A meta-analysis of homeopathic clinical trials published in the *The Lancet* in 1997 by Klaus Linde, M.D., examined nearly ninety well-designed, randomized clinical trials. The combined results from all these studies also tended to support homeopathy. In addition to studies reporting homeopathy's effectiveness, there are also those that report its limitations. Dr. Pelletier, for example, points to studies that show that homeopathy is *unsuccessful* in treating plantar warts and osteoarthritis and in *preventing* illness. Both Dr. Pelletier and Dr. Linde stress the need for more well-designed studies of homeopathy.[28]

4

HEADACHES
AND MIGRAINES

*N*ote that severe head pain associated with a stiff neck, drowsiness or pinpoint rash may be a symptom of meningitis, a life-threatening condition that requires a trip to the emergency room of a hospital. Please see Chapter 8, "Belly Problems," and Chapter 10, "Bumps, Bruises, Burns, Cuts and Pain in Bones and Muscles," for descriptions of other pain in children that requires immediate attention.

When serious causes of head pain are ruled out, sometimes what is diagnosed as either tension headaches or migraines is the result of chronic tight muscles in the head and neck, says Joy Weydert, M.D., FAAP, director of Integrative Pain

Management at Children's Mercy Hospital in Kansas City. "These tight muscles may be the result of physical or emotional trauma, or anything that causes stress on the nervous system," says Weydert. "We see a lot of kids who come in with this kind of pain, and for many it is the result of tension they are experiencing at school. In fact, some kids see headache pain as an avenue for getting out of school."

Is It a Tension Headache or Not?

If a headache does not improve with rest, medication or the integrative methods mentioned below, or if it wakes a child up at night or happens first thing in the morning, have your child evaluated by a doctor. The cause may be something other than stress, especially if the headache is accompanied by visual or hearing problems. But because headaches and stress are so closely linked, you should also explore what kind of stress your child may be under at home or at school, and try to figure out ways to alleviate that stress.

For tension or migraine headaches, Dr. Weydert recommends:

- *Insure proper hydration.* Encourage several glasses of water daily, and substitute water for soda!
- *Improve sleep habits with good wake/sleep cycles.* (See Chapter 9, "I Can't Sleep.")
- *Craniosacral therapy/osteopathic manipulation therapy.* (See "A Closer Look at Osteopathy and Craniosacral Therapy.")
- *Magnesium supplements* (in the form of glycinate, gluconate, aspartate, oxide). This is a natural muscle relaxant and pain reliever. The recommended dosage is 250 to 500 milligrams orally twice a day, but **always consult with your pediatrician.**
- *Massage therapy.* (See "A Closer Look at Massage for Children.")
- *Breathing and relaxation techniques, guided imagery.* (See guidelines in Chapter 2.)
- *Biofeedback.*
- *Acupuncture/acupressure.*
- *Herbal foot baths or compresses.* Your child might enjoy a special foot bath! Use warm or cold baths, whichever is more comfortable for your child. You can also alternate warm and cold baths using the calming botanicals listed below.

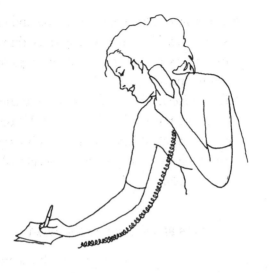

- *Botanicals.* **(Always consult with your pediatrician before giving these to your child.)**

  - *Ginger root capsules, tea or extracts.* Ginger opens small blood vessels, has anti-inflammatory effects and relieves nausea. Take three to four times a day orally following package dosing instructions.
  - *Feverfew.* This herb relieves minor pain and muscle spasms. Take as extract or capsules three to four times a day orally following package dosing instructions. Use whole herb products.

- *Chamomile*. This herb is calming and antispasmodic. Take as tea or extract three to four times a day orally following package dosing instructions.
- *Lemon balm*. This herb has calming effects. It can be taken orally as tea or 1-2 drops of the essential oil can be diluted with 1 tsp. of vegetable oil and applied to the skin where there is pain.

Bumps and Bruises to the Head

If your child has a head injury, call the doctor if there is loss of consciousness, a decreased level of consciousness or if there is vomiting more than once. If your child falls asleep after the injury, wake her up every thirty minutes to make sure she is still alert. Nonserious head bumps can be treated in the same way as other bodily injuries. (See Chapter 10, "Bumps, Bruises, Burns, Cuts and Pain in Bones and Muscles.")

5

TEETHING PROBLEMS

This is a small chapter about a big problem. Teething pain is hard for both child and parent. Your child is suffering, yet conventional medicine offers little help. We've all tried the teething biscuits, frozen Popsicles and pacifiers, as well as the over-the-counter remedies, with varying degrees of success. Here are some integrative suggestions from Joy A. Weydert, M.D., FAAP, director of Integrative Pain Management at Children's Mercy Hospital in Kansas City.

- *Herbal tea made with chamomile.* Steep 1 teaspoon in 1 cup hot water for ten minutes, then strain and cool. Give 1 ounce every few hours.

- *Homeopathic remedies.* **(Consult with your pediatrician and/or homeopathic physician before using.)** Suggested remedies include chamomilla, belladonna, calcarea carbonica/phosphorica, silicea—used alone or in combination.
- *Clove essential oil.* Dilute 1 to 2 drops in 1 teaspoon of vegetable oil and apply with cotton swab to sore gums.
- *Aromatherapy.* Use calming essential oils such as lavender, chamomile or lemon balm. Dilute 3 to 5 drops in bathwater or add to 2 tablespoons of vegetable oil before applying topically with massage on the skin. **Test this first on a small area of skin for one hour to check for any sensitivity before applying extensively. Never give essential oils internally or apply undiluted directly to the skin.**

6

COLDS AND FEVER

The herbal remedies, saltwater nose rinse and anti-inflammatory food suggestions for asthma and upper respiratory infections described in Chapter 2 are also useful in the treatment of colds and fever in children. But there is one healing system that we have not yet mentioned: European Natural Medicine. This is a system based on stimulating the body's natural healing ability through acknowledging our innate biological heritage: Like our cave ancestors, our bodies perform best when they are exercised, exposed to fresh air, and consume a diet based on freshness and the whole foods that have evolved with us for millions of years. Our expert on this subject is Alexa

Fleckenstein, M.D., a board-certified internist with a subspecialty in European Natural Medicine and the author of the forthcoming book, *Health by Water* (Contemporary Books, in press). While Dr. Fleckenstein is not a pediatrician, many of the healing methods she uses to treat colds and fever in adult patients are also appropriate for children.

Preventing the Common Cold

To prevent colds, Dr. Fleckenstein suggests teaching children from a very young age to wash hands frequently and to cover their mouths when coughing or sneezing. Going out every day—no matter what the weather—stimulates and strengthens the immune system. "As long as children are bundled up appropriately against the weather, there is no reason not to be outside," says Dr. Fleckenstein, who is a native of Germany and grew up with a tradition of walking, hiking and outdoor activities.

Treating Colds and Fever

I do not recommend over-the-counter cold medications, including decongestants, cough syrups or antihistamines. Studies have shown that while you may get some relief, these medicines are not very effective for colds and the side effects outweigh the benefits. Decongestants and antihistamines alleviate the symptoms only marginally or not at all, and they hinder the immune system as it works to heal your child; they might also increase the clogging by drying the sinus contents.

Because aspirin is contraindicated in children, acetaminophen (Tylenol) or ibuprofen are usually recommended as fever-reducing agents. But by lowering the body temperature, you hinder the body's natural mechanism for slowing or killing viruses and bacteria. If you do decide to lower the fever, in consultation with your pediatrician, consider trying the nonmedication methods listed below before resorting to medication. *Of course, you should always call your pediatrician if your child has a severe sore throat, a fever of 103 degrees or over, or prolonged fever (three days or more), or anything else that worries you.*

If a cold strikes, Dr. Fleckenstein's home-care program is a good way to begin caring for your child, and the sooner the better. "The earlier you treat a cold, the less likely that it will develop into a full-blown infection for which you have to see the doctor," she says. Here are her treatment recommendations, combining conventional care with methods derived from European Natural Medicine:

- *Rest.* This cold is telling the body something. "It takes two to get sick," says Dr. Fleckenstein, "a virus and a run-down immune system. So let your child rest as much as possible, and aim for early bedtimes."
- *Rinse your child's nose with salt water* with the first signs of stuffed or running nose. The common cold starts in the upper nose, leads to swelling of the nasal mucosa, and only then to clogging of the sinuses and the ears (eustachian tubes). Later it can run down the trachea (breathing tube) and cause bronchitis and pneumonia. So try to stop this process early. See instructions for sinus irrigation in Chapter 3. You can use this method starting at about age eight; for younger children, use an eyedropper to put a few drops of the saltwater solution into your child's nostril to unclog the nose.

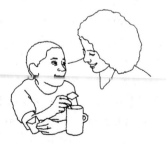

- *Hot fluids.* Hot water, hot broth (chicken soup has been researched—and it really works!), hot herbal teas (linden flowers, elderberry flowers, honeysuckle, fennel or thyme) are good—and so are many others. Hot lemonade is also beneficial, made with fresh lemons and preferably without honey or sugar.

- *Respect your child's appetite.* Do not force your child to eat if he is not hungry. Avoid refined sugar, starches and dairy (since dairy may thicken mucus). If your child wants to eat, encourage food made with garlic and onions, or leeks and shallots.

- *Hot blueberry soup.* Barely cover the contents of one package of frozen blueberries with water; bring to a fast boil, then allow to cool enough for the child to eat the whole concoction of berries and liquid. This gives your child vitamins and minerals to help fight infection. And the blue color in the blueberries kills infectious agents, too. (By the way, this soup is also good for acute stomach flu and urinary tract infections.) Hot elderberry soup is good, too—but hard to come by. You can buy the elderberry juice as Sambucol® (but blueberries are much cheaper).

- *Herbs.* In addition to the herbs listed in

previous chapters, children over the age of three can be given extracts of *Echinacea angustifolia* root, olive leaf, pau d'arco and osha. **Check with your pediatrician first, and do not use for more than one week without the approval of your doctor.**

- *Gargle* with salt water or warm water (mix a teaspoon of salt in eight ounces of water with 1 drop of sage or myrrh). **This should not be done by children under the age of six.**

- *Steam inhalation* helps with a running or stuffed nose. You can add chamomile, eucalyptus or a tiny piece of Vicks VapoRub Ointment. You can also use Vicks on older children (check the label).

- *Acupuncture* helps with a cold, but may be costly. Says Dr. Fleckenstein: "I would give it a try if you are looking for more immediate results. Otherwise, view this cold as a necessary down time for both you and your child."

Sore Throat

- *Herbs that soothe* sore throats include slippery elm, marshmallow root and licorice. **Use as teas in consultation with your pediatrician.**

- *Zinc lozenges*. One zinc gluconate lozenge up

to four times a day might help a sore throat—
but find a sugar-free, acid-free brand.

Cough

Coughs due to acute inflammation or chronic
bronchitis are treated with the following soothing
herbs, used in teas. Cough syrups are not effective
and I do not recommend them. *Use the following
herbs in consultation with your pediatrician.*

- Marshmallow root *(Althea officinalis)*
- Slippery elm bark *(Ulmus fulva)*
- Mullein flowers *(Verbascum spp.)*
- The juice of plantain *(Plantago lanceolata/
  silicic acid)*

High Fever

For high fevers—over 103 degrees—that do not
respond to the treatments mentioned above, keep
encouraging fluids, and, in consultation with your
doctor, try acetaminophen or ibuprofen.

A CLOSER LOOK

Acupuncture and Traditional Chinese Medicine (TCM): Restoring the Flow

Integrative pediatrician Lawrence Rosen, M.D., grew up going to conventional doctors, but as a very young boy he learned about other methods of healing from his grandfather. "My grandfather emigrated to the United States from Eastern Europe and was interested in non-Western cultures," says Dr. Rosen. "He was particularly fascinated by Native American and Far Eastern traditions, and he introduced me to the concept of the Native American medicine man. His stories fascinated me, and I learned from him about healing within the circle of life and nature. That philosophy stayed with me all through medical school."

After Dr. Rosen graduated and became a pediatrician, he became frustrated with the limitations of conventional Western medicine. "The system that I learned in medical school is great for treating acute illnesses and injuries, but is less effective for many of the chronic pediatric problems I was seeing, including allergies, autism, chronic abdominal pain, headaches, irritable bowel syndrome and attention deficit/hyperactivity disorder (ADHD)." So Dr. Rosen embarked on a mission to learn more about alternative healing methods, apprenticing himself to experts in Traditional Chinese Medicine (TCM), homeopathy and nutrition and becoming trained in mind/body techniques such as biofeedback and guided imagery. He now has a holistic, integrative pediatric practice, regularly referring his young patients for acupuncture and offering massage, Reiki energy work, biofeedback, herbal medicine and mind/body practices for pediatric problems. He also directs the Integrative Pediatric Service at the Maria Fareri Children's Hospital in Westchester County, New York.

An important part of Dr. Rosen's practice involves introducing and explaining alternative practices to parents. "Traditional Chinese Medicine, for example, is a complete and ancient healing medical system that understands the body as a whole unit: Every organ and tissue has a relationship to every other, to the body as a whole, to the mind and emotions and also to the environment and even the universe," says Dr. Rosen. "Western medicine understands the body only in relation to itself, and usually sees organs, bones, muscles and limbs as isolated units, which is of course useful in the diagnosis and treatment of trauma and acute problems, but limited in the treatment of chronic conditions."

Another explanation of Traditional Chinese

Medicine comes from Dr. Cheng Xiao Ming, who trained in Western orthopedic surgery in China and then went back to school for a second medical degree in Traditional Chinese Medicine. Thanks to many years of teaching acupuncture and other Chinese healing methods to American students in Boston, Dr. Cheng is accustomed to explaining TCM philosophy and theory to the Western mind. "I ask my students, 'Who lives longer, the rabbit or the turtle?' They all answer, 'The turtle, of course,'" Dr. Cheng says. "Then I ask them, 'So does this mean we should all live like turtles?' 'Of course not!' they say. 'We'd never get anywhere.'"

At this point, his eyes twinkle. "Then I say to them, 'On the outside, we should be like a rabbit, strengthening our muscles, exercising our bodies and running when we need to. But on the inside, we should be like a turtle, breathing slowly and deeply, slowing the heart when it is at rest, creating a peaceful internal environment. Just like we have to train our bodies to be strong, we must also train our minds and internal organs to relax. When you are peaceful, you can logically and calmly resolve any problem, even if there is turmoil around you.'" This rabbit and turtle story appeals to young children and helps them understand the TCM philosophy and how it relates to their own health.

One way for children (and adults) to attain a

peaceful internal environment is through Traditional Chinese Medicine exercises—known as "qigong" and "tai chi," which are slow, graceful movements that help to slow down the mind and move qi (universal energy, pronounced "chi") inside the body. By changing the inner environment of the body, both of these forms of exercise are thought to improve the actual functions of organs and tissues. Even children as young as six can benefit from the focused meditative skills they learn in tai chi or qigong classes, says Dr. Rosen. "Older children might particularly respond to qigong, which, despite its slow, dancelike qualities, did originate with a martial arts focus."

It is the flow of qi along pathways called "meridians" inside the body that is the focus of all Chinese medical treatments. Even though meridians are invisible, thousands of years of practice and observation have resulted in clearly mapped diagrams of their routes within the body. Most practitioners of Chinese medicine have large drawings on the walls of their offices showing the elaborate network of meridians throughout the body. If you have ever had acupuncture and felt the tingling sensation along a meridian when a tiny needle is inserted into just the right spot, you would think that the meridians must indeed be as visible and tangible as your blood vessels. "The needles don't cure disease," explains Dr. Cheng. "They adjust the qi energy, reinforcing it, reducing it where necessary, moving stagnant or 'stuck' energy. With the free flow of energy restored, the body can heal itself. After all, our bodies fight off viruses and bacteria every day. TCM methods increase that ability."

Other TCM methods include the use of Chinese herbs, taken internally or put directly on the skin, deep tissue massage (called *tui na*), and qigong massage (during which the practitioner uses the hands to transmit and move qi energy with the patient fully clothed). Like other integrative pediatricians, Dr. Rosen believes in combining alternative methods from such systems as TCM with conventional Western treatments for his patients. "The integrative approach may use Western diagnostic methods and TCM or other alternative treatments," says Dr. Rosen. But there are even differences in diagnosis: Western medicine diagnoses and treats a disease. TCM diagnoses by symptom, using more than twelve different wrist pulses, the condition of the tongue, and palpation (feeling) muscles and other tissues along meridians.

Dr. Cheng describes the youngest patient he has ever treated: The baby was only eight weeks old

and diagnosed with a life-threatening form of diarrhea. Antibiotics were tried but could not stop the
near-constant diarrhea. "The mother brought me
her baby," says Dr. Cheng. "I used tui na massage as
well as acupuncture and taught the mother to perform the massage at home." The treatments slowed
and then stopped the diarrhea, and the child is now
a healthy six-year-old.

Many problems diagnosed in Chinese medicine
are said to relate to imbalance between *yin* and
yang energy in the body. Yin energy is represented
by the more "quiet" characteristics of organs and
structures in the body. It nourishes the inside of the
body. Yang energy is more active, causing change or
activity. "You can't have one without the other,"
says Dr. Cheng. "A car, for example, can't run (yang
activity) without the gas (yin nourishment). For
good health, the yin and yang energies need to be
in harmonious balance."

TCM for Children

The following information is from Dr. Lawrence Rosen's excellent Web site about integrative medicine for children (*www.thewholechild.us*):

"Traditional Chinese Medicine (TCM) is a whole system of healing based on holistic philosophies involving balance of yin and yang, natural elements of earth, metal, water, fire and wood, mind-body-spirit harmony, and the flow of qi, blood, and moisture. . . . Practitioners in the West have long adopted certain TCM methods like acupuncture for very specific conditions, like pain; yet TCM in its true form does not utilize acupuncture piecemeal, nor does it only use one method for each condition or patient. Other TCM healing measures include:

- Tui na (massage), which can be tailored specifically for infants and children
- Herbal remedies, which are complex mixtures of animals, plants and minerals; manufacturer Kan Herbs has trustworthy, specific formulations for children, and, as with all botanicals, one must be cognizant of quality control issues—some imported Ayurvedic and TCM products have been contaminated with lead

and other metals, as well as mislabeled herbs.
- Qi gong and tai chi, both of which are movement-based disciplines aimed at supporting mind/body wellness.
- Nutrition and other lifestyle considerations."

TCM: Ancient Wisdom for Modern Times

Traditional Chinese Medicine is a well-developed, coherent system of medicine that has been practiced in China for thousands of years. "As an extensive and established medical system, TCM is used by billions of people around the world for every condition known to humankind," writes Lixing Lao, Ph.D., L.Ac., associate professor in the Department of Complementary Medicine, University of Maryland School of Medicine.[29] There are hundreds of research studies documenting the effectiveness of Traditional Chinese Medicine for children and adults. But Lao notes that perhaps the most poetic citation comes not from the modern research literature, but from *The Yellow Emperor's Classic of Internal Medicine*, thought to be the first classic work on Traditional Chinese Medicine, published 300 BC:

> *In a peaceful calm,*
> *Void and emptiness,*
> *The authentic Qi*
> *Flows easily.*
> *Essences and spirits*
> *Are kept within.*
> *How could illness arise?*

WHAT'S THE EVIDENCE?

TCM for Specific Childhood Problems

Because of the mind/body approach of TCM, this ancient medical system can be used for most childhood illnesses, says Lawrence Rosen, M.D. If you worry about your child's reaction to the tiny acupuncture needles, consider a study at Children's Hospital in Boston.[30] "In this study, young children with chronic pain were offered acupuncture as part of their treatment, and most reported great improvement," says Dr. Rosen. "The needles are tiny and relatively painless, but if children really object to needles, the same benefits can be obtained by using acupressure—massage of the acupuncture points—as well as the use of lasers on the acupuncture points."

Research has shown that acupuncture is effective in children for a variety of problems,[31] including:

- Post-operative pain
- Stomach pain
- Nausea and vomiting (especially during chemotherapy)
- Muscle, joint and bone pain
- Fibromyalgia
- Migraine and other headaches

Movement therapies such as qigong and tai chi can help children with these conditions as well as those with attention deficit/hyperactivity disorder (ADHD). "The focus and concentration they learn while studying these movements translates into other areas of their lives," says Dr. Rosen. In addition, Dr. Rosen and his colleagues are studying the effectiveness of TCM and other alternative/complementary treatments for children with autism.

7

COLIC

One of my colleagues has two children, both of whom had bouts of colic that lasted for several months after birth. The babies would wail and cry miserably almost nonstop from about 8 P.M. until midnight. Their legs were drawn up toward their abdomens and their faces were flushed. The pediatrician had little advice other than to recommend that the nursing mother avoid eating spicy food, so the exhausted parents spent every night walking and rocking the baby. There was no lasting damage; both kids had happy, otherwise healthy childhoods and are now flourishing in college. But I wish these parents had known twenty years ago about the following suggested integrative remedies from Dr. Joy Weydert:

- *Herbal teas made with chamomile, fennel, lemon balm, ginger.* Use one or a combination, steep 1 teaspoon in 1 cup hot water for ten minutes, then strain and cool. Give 1 ounce every few hours.
- *Gripe Water.* This is an herbal extract typically made with dill, caraway, cinnamon bark oil, cardamom and cloves, and it is given orally. **Use only nonalcohol extracts** and follow packaging instructions. Colic-Ease is one brand manufactured in FDA-approved laboratories. This product can be found in health food stores or on the Internet. **Consult with your pediatrician first.**
- *Cranial osteopathy and craniosacral therapy.* (See "A Closer Look at Osteopathy and Craniosacral Therapy.")
- *Infant massage.* (See "A Closer Look at Massage for Children.")
- *Homeopathic remedies.* **Always consult first with your pediatrician or a homeopathic physician.** Use chamomilla, colocynthis, magnesia phosphorica—alone or in combination.

- *Aromatherapy.* You can use essential oils of lavender, chamomile, lemon balm or other calming herbs. Dilute 3 to 5 drops in bath water or add to 2 tablespoons of vegetable oil before applying topically with gentle massage. **Test this first on a small area of skin for one hour to check for any sensitivity before applying extensively. Never give essential oils internally or apply undiluted directly to the skin.**

- *Acupressure.* This is a form of Traditional Chinese Medicine that should be performed by a certified professional. (See "A Closer Look at Acupuncture and Traditional Chinese Medicine.")

- *Probiotics: acidophilus, lactobacillus, bifidus, Saccharomyces boulardii.* Probiotics are considered "beneficial bacteria" used to restore the normal flora of the intestines to improve digestion. These are especially important if the child has received antibiotics in the past. *Ask your pediatrician* where to buy these and for dosage recommendations.

- *Breastfeeding moms.* Decrease or eliminate gas-forming foods, as well as citrus, milk, caffeine and chocolate, as these cross over through breast milk.

- *In addition*, use swaddling, holding, warm baths, gentle rocking and womb noises.

This too shall pass: Remember that colic usually doesn't last more than a few months. You *will* sleep again!

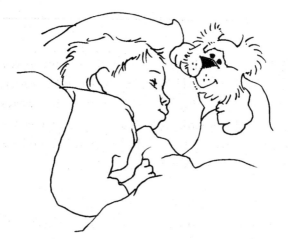

8

BELLY PROBLEMS:
"I HAVE A STOMACHACHE!"

I f your child is complaining about pain in the belly that is sudden (acute onset) and is associated with vomiting and no appetite, or if it wakes your child up from sleep, go to the emergency room. Belly problems that require immediate medical attention include:

- Appendicitis.
- Intussusception: This condition, which usually occurs in infants, is the telescoping inward of the bowel usually after a viral infection. It usually starts near where the small bowel turns into the large bowel and causes

the intestines to fold inward like a telescope. It is thought to occur as the result of inflamed lymph nodes.

• Volvulus: twisted intestine.

If there is chronic pain with no relief, ask your pediatrician to check the child. Acute and persistent belly problems that require ongoing doctor supervision include Crohn's disease, ulcerative colitis, inflammatory bowel syndrome and celiac disease. While some of these can benefit from alternative therapies, as we describe in this book, you should always work in consultation with your pediatrician.

After your pediatrician has ruled out appendicitis and all other acute abdominal problems, you might consider two lifestyle issues that may negatively affect your child's digestion: stress and diet. Ever wonder why you get intestinal cramps or "butterflies in the stomach" when you are nervous? In the embryonic stage, the gut develops from the same tissue as the brain, so it makes sense that there is an intimate connection between the brain and the belly. There are as many nerve fibers in the intestine as in the central nervous system. The "sympathetic nervous system," which responds to your emotions and to stress, can cause pain in the belly and problems with digestion.

A SECOND BRAIN IN THE GUT? EVIDENCE SAYS YES

In addition to the brain and central nervous system we all know about, there is evidence that a second complex "brain" and nervous system also exist in the human gut. The gut brain, called the enteric nervous system, has been described by Michael Gershon, M.D., professor of anatomy and cell biology at Columbia Presbyterian Medical Center in New York. In a 1996 interview with the *New York Times,* Dr. Gershon explained that nearly every substance that helps run and control the brain has turned up in the gut. These include serotonin, dopamine, glutamate, norephinephrine and nitric oxide, as well as two dozen small brain proteins, called neuropeptides, and major cells of the immune system.[32]

Dr. Gershon is considered one of the founders of a new field of medicine called neurogastroenterology. More information and research is available from the International Foundation for Functional Gastrointestinal Disorders *(www. iffgd.org)*, as well as the University of North Carolina Division of Digestive Diseases *(www.med.unc.edu/medicine/gi)*.

Because of the intimate connection between the brain and the gut, even very young children can experience belly pain and digestive problems that are related to stress or anxiety. Joy Weydert, M.D., director of Integrative Pain Management at Children's Mercy Hospital, describes a six-year-old girl with persistent belly pain with no obvious physical cause. "I taught this little girl some breathing and relaxation techniques, which she practiced at home with her parents," says Dr. Weydert. "After four weeks, her belly pain was all but gone, and she had taught the techniques to her older cousin, who used them to help reduce headache pain."

TEACH YOUR CHILD TO RELAX

Here are some of the breathing and relaxation techniques suggested by Joy Weydert, M.D. They can be used with children as young as three.

BREATHING EXERCISES

With very young children, begin by using a bubble wand to teach them how to control their breath well enough to

she points out. That she has come to this conclusion as a pediatrician is significant because Dr. Weydert grew up on a farm. "I had ice cream and milk every day growing up," she says. "I was also always congested and had sinus problems, as well as having trouble with digestion. When I became an adult, I stopped eating dairy products, except for the very occasional taste of cheese or yogurt, which I think are more easily digested. My congestion, sinus and digestive problems have cleared up completely. Cow's milk, I believe, is seen by the body as a foreign protein and may contribute to chronic ear infections, asthma, sinus infections, congestion and digestive problems for many kids."

Other possible inflammatory foods include anything that is processed, including cookies, packaged snacks and anything made with partially hydrogenated oils; anything, in fact, with a long shelf life. Better to fill your child's diet with fresh fruit, vegetables, whole grains and other high fiber foods. Don't forget to include healthful fats—especially omega 3, which is in cold-water fish, flaxseed oil, walnuts and other nuts. Instead of a cookie jar, keep a big jar of nuts, raisins and other dried fruit on the counter. You can also give your children flax oil supplements in smoothies and sprinkle flaxseed on salads. If you are worried about your kids getting enough calcium if they don't eat dairy foods, give them soy milk; calcium-fortified orange juice; plenty of green, leafy vegetables; and beans and nuts.

Food Summary for Digestive Problems

Avoid:

- Any processed foods and anything made with hydrogenated and partially hydrogenated oils, including cookies, crackers, snacks.
- Anything with a long shelf life.
- Bread or baked goods made with white flour.
- White sugar (difficult—but do the best you can!).
- Cow's milk may contribute to chronic ear infections, asthma, sinus infections, congestion and digestive problems for many children. To test this idea, eliminate cow's milk from your child's diet for two weeks and see what happens.

Encourage your child to eat:

- Fresh vegetables
- Fresh fruit
- Whole grains
- Cold-water fish

- Flaxseed oil
- Walnuts and other nuts
- Snacks from a cookie jar filled with a mixture of raisins, dried fruit and nuts

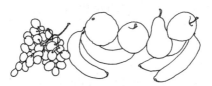

Gastro-Esophageal Reflux Disease (GERD)

This is a problem we are seeing more and more of in babies and young children. The contents of the stomach come up into the esophagus, causing spitting up and discomfort. This condition may be caused by stress and also by diets too high in saturated fat. I recommend lower-fat diets, stress reduction through the breathing and relaxation techniques described in this chapter, and manual therapies such as craniosacral therapy. (See "A Closer Look at Osteopathy and Craniosacral Therapy.") Be careful of antispasmodic herbs—such as mint or chamomile—or some dietary supplements because they can increase GERD symptoms.

Treating Belly Pain

After you have ruled out acute, serious problems, **consult with your pediatrician** about the following:

- *Eliminate possible food allergens/intolerances*, such as milk, dairy products and processed foods with a long shelf life.
- *Encourage healthful eating.*
- *Give the child probiotics (acidophilus, lactobacillus, bifidobacterium, saccharomyces)* to restore natural intestinal balance, especially if the child has been on antibiotics. **Always consult with your pediatrician.**
- *"Hands-on" manual therapy* such as:
  - *Abdominal massage.* (See "A Closer Look at Massage for Children.")
  - *Breathing/relaxation techniques.* (See sidebar "Teach Your Child to Relax" in this chapter.)
  - *Guided imagery, biofeedback.* (See sidebar "Teaching Guided Imagery and Visualization to Children" in Chapter 2.)
  - *Acupuncture/acupressure.* (See "A Closer Look at Acupuncture and Traditional Chinese Medicine.")
- *Botanicals that soothe the stomach and intestines. Check with your pediatrician before giving these to your child:*

- *Chamomile* is calming and antispasmodic. Give as tea or extract three to four times a day orally following package instructions. Do not use for GERD as it may make the condition worse.
- *Slippery elm* coats inflamed tissues and ulcers and can be given as a tea or extract three to four times a day orally following package dosing instructions.
- *Deglycyrrhizinated licorice* coats irritated tissues and ulcers and is also anti-inflammatory. It is good for heartburn symptoms. It comes in chewable tablets taken orally following package instructions.
- *Enteric-coated peppermint* is an antispasmodic digestive agent that is good for lower abdominal symptoms. It comes in tablets that are taken orally two to three times a day. Do not use with GERD as it may make the condition worse.
- *Marshmallow root* coats irritated tissues and ulcers and supports your child's immune system. It can be taken orally as a tea, an extract or capsules two to three times a day.
- *Ginger* opens small blood vessels, has anti-inflammatory effects and relieves nausea. It

can be taken orally as capsules, tea or extracts three to four times a day following package instructions.

A CLOSER LOOK

Massage for Children

A researcher's determination to help her own infant was the beginning of therapeutic massage—also known as touch therapy—as a medical treatment in this country. With the birth of her premature daughter, Tiffany Field, Ph.D., looked for ways to help her thrive and gain weight. "She massaged her daughter daily and found that this practice reduced the infant's anxiety, encouraged her to take more formula and helped her gain weight. This led Dr. Field to hypothesize that similar and additional improvements might be observed in other premature infants if they were massaged in a similar manner."[33]

Massage involves touch and movement. It is "the systematic manipulation of the soft tissues of the body to enhance health and healing."[34] Dr. Field tested her hypothesis in several clinical trials, finding that premature infants who were massaged grew and developed better than those who were not massaged. She has since gone on to perform massage therapy research for other conditions and is now director of the Touch Research Institute at the University of Miami School of Medicine (*www. miami.edu/touch-research*). Of course, the practice of massage in this country was going on long before Dr. Field began her research. Dr. Linda Freeman summarizes the highlights:

In the nineteenth century, two physicians and brothers brought the Swedish Movement Cure to the United States, using their techniques to stimulate skin, muscle, blood vessels, the lymph system, nerves and some internal organs.[35] The first massage therapy clinics in the United States were opened by the Swedes after the Civil War. During the first part of the twentieth century, Swedish massage became popular at private health clubs, hospitals and with professional sports teams. The practice declined during the 1940s and 1950s, coming back into prominence during the holistic health and healing movements of the Sixties and the wellness movement that began in the Seventies.

"This led health professionals to reevaluate the therapeutic value of touch and massage. The American Nurses Association recognized massage therapy as an official nursing subspecialty, and therapeutic touch, an energy form of healing, was warmly embraced by nursing professionals. Of greatest impact was the growing number of massage therapists performing massage and body work full-time."[36] In some European countries, such as Germany, massage is considered part of conventional medicine.

Learning Infant Massage

There are several excellent Web sites, books and videos that teach you how to do infant massage. For example, the Web site *http://babiestoday.com* gives detailed instructions on massage for upset stomachs and fussy babies, including belly massage and foot massage. (See Resources at the end of this book for books offering instructions with photos and illustrations on how to perform baby massage.)

Ancient Traditions for Modern Times

Massage therapy has been a health practice of most ancient cultures, including China, India, Persia, Arabia and Greece. Hippocrates used massage to treat sprains and dislocations, Aristotle treated exhaustion by massaging the body with oil and water, and oil massage was used in Sparta and Athens in preparation for vigorous exercise. Descriptions of tui na and acupressure appeared in the pages of *The Yellow Emperor's Classic of Internal*

Medicine, written about 300 BC and believed to be the first book of Chinese medicine. Indian Ayurvedic massage practices date back to the fifth century BC. The recent revival of infant massage in this country has been patterned on the ancient practice of Indian baby massage.[37]

WHAT'S THE EVIDENCE?

Massage

Dr. Tiffany Field's research found that premature newborns who received massage therapy showed greater growth, weight gain, and improved cognitive and motor development at eight months than non-massaged infants.[38] Since that time, research from randomized controlled studies suggests positive effects of massage for anxiety and premenstrual syndrome. For patients with fibromyalgia, it has been suggested to relieve pain and depression and improve the quality of life. It also was found to have potential for the treatment of both lower back pain and chronic constipation.[39] However, another review of massage therapy reported that "evidence to support massage as a treatment to promote development in preterm and/or low birthweight infants is weak."[40]

But aside from the research, any parent knows that a loving touch can make almost anything feel better! Children with juvenile rheumatoid arthritis (one of the most common chronic diseases of childhood) were massaged by their parents for fifteen minutes each night. Another group practiced relaxation with their parents for the same amount of time. At the end of thirty days, both the parents and children in the massage group experienced lower anxiety (determined by behavioral observation and levels of cortisol, a stress hormone, in the saliva). The massaged children reported significantly less pain after massage and fewer pain episodes than the relaxation group.[41] Massage therapy also decreased the number of migraine headaches and reduced sleep disturbances and related distress symptoms.[42]

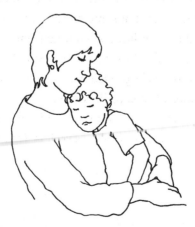

9

"I CAN'T SLEEP"

Many childhood health problems, whether related to headache, belly pain, indigestion or the muscle aches of fibromyalgia, can be improved if your child can get a good night's sleep. Sleep is restorative. It is during sleep that our bodies make growth hormones, repair damaged cells and reduce pain. For some children, insomnia may be a medical condition stemming from a variety of factors, including stress, medications for ADHD, illness or poor sleep hygiene. Here is a story from Joy Weydert, M.D., to illustrate:

The patient was a young man of seventeen with such a severe case of fibromyalgia (overall body aches and pains and fatigue) that he could barely move, eat or sleep. He could not attend school and was understandably miserable. Dr. Weydert, director of Integrative Pain Management, was called in to see him after he had been hospitalized at Children's Mercy Hospital for the pain. "Even narcotics did nothing to help him," says Dr. Weydert. "He had been in and out of the hospital for months, and at this point, they had to insert a feeding tube for nourishment because he was in too much pain to eat." This young man did not believe in the value of alternative medicine, so at first was not receptive to Dr. Weydert's suggestions of massage therapy, guided imagery, breathing or relaxation techniques.

"But after some time at home with the feeding tube and finding little relief from the narcotics, he came back to the clinic nearly in tears, ready to at least listen to my suggestions," says Dr. Weydert. "It is important to meet kids where they are and only offer them what you feel they can accept. So I began with an herbal tea mixture that I use to help kids sleep because I felt that, as a first step, he needed to get some rest." The boy took the tea home on a Friday, after first suspiciously asking Dr. Weydert, "Is this legal?" On Monday morning, his mother called to say that he had slept well for the first time in months. "This was the open door I needed," says Dr. Weydert. "After that, he agreed to other therapies to reduce the pain, including massage and craniosacral therapy. Finally, he also agreed to acupuncture, which he later described as the turning point in his recovery."

The combination worked, and he was soon eating well and back at school. When he had a recent flare-up of pain, Dr. Weydert diagnosed trigger points, which are tight muscle segments that press on nerves and sent him for a more conventional treatment—trigger point injections that numb the area enough to let the muscles relax. "With more time, alternative techniques like massage, craniosacral therapy and the Alexander Technique (which teaches people to use their bodies with less effort) would have helped as well, but he needed immediate relief, so we used a conventional method," says Dr. Weydert. "But the beauty and effectiveness of integrative medicine is that we— and our patients—have a larger array of treatment choices."

DR. JOY WEYDERT'S
RELAXING HERBAL TEA

This combination of herbs is what Dr. Weydert uses to help children get a good night's sleep: chamomile, lemon balm, hops, valerian, hibiscus, lavender, skullcap, dalmation sage, thyme, rosemary, passion flower and spearmint. Most of these are available as teas in health food stores. If you can't find a ready-made blend with a combination of these herbs, Dr. Weydert suggests choosing two or three from the list to mix together in equal parts and store in an airtight container. Use one teaspoon of the mix to make one cup of tea. Always consult with your pediatrician before giving your child herbs.

How to Help Your Child Sleep

After you and your doctor have evaluated and treated such insomnia causes as medication, pain or illness, here are suggestions for good sleep hygiene: At least an hour before bedtime, turn off anything that is too stimulating—such as TV, computers and video games. Avoid giving children anything that contains caffeine, including chocolate. Begin to turn the lights down or off in the house. Dimmer lights induce the production of melatonin in the brain, which is a chemical that makes us sleepy. This is our evolutionary heritage from ancestors who went to sleep as the sun went down because they did not have electricity! With too much artificial light at the end of the day, the brain does not receive the signal that it is time to slow down. In fact, studies of people who work night shifts and therefore have disrupted melatonin production show that such people are more prone to cancer. Disrupted sleep has also been linked to obesity.

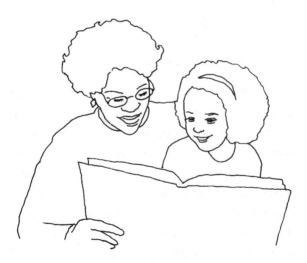

So the hour before bedtime should be a time of dim lights, perhaps quiet music or reading stories, and a calming herbal tea. (See sidebar for Dr. Weydert's recipe.) One parent I know would pretend to sprinkle fairy dust over her very young children when they were in bed to help them fall asleep and have happy dreams. (Whatever works!)

10

BUMPS, BRUISES,
BURNS, CUTS AND PAIN
IN BONES AND MUSCLES

We have all heard (and probably used) the expression, "It's just growing pains." And while our children certainly are growing, and may experience unexplained pain, there are certain bone and muscle pains that should not be ignored. I once had a four-year-old patient whose only complaint was pain in one leg when she walked. There was no swelling, no bruising and nothing to indicate a cause. One round of blood tests was normal, but still she complained. It would have been easy to dismiss this as a "growing pain," but I was not satisfied. A four-year-old should not be complaining of this kind of pain. We repeated the blood tests and found an abnormally low white blood count (hemoglobin and platelets were normal). It was leukemia, but it was still in the bone marrow and had not made it into the bloodstream yet. We had caught it early enough for an effective treatment. She is a teenager now and doing wonderfully.

Be suspicious of any bone, joint or muscle pain that persists, and get medical attention for your child, repeating tests if necessary.

Under the age of two, children express pain through irritability or screaming if you touch or move a part of their bodies that hurts. Following a cold, infants can develop an infection in the bloodstream that can seep into any joint—especially the hip joint—that could destroy the joint or cause death. In this situation, the baby will be irritable or scream if you touch or move an arm or a leg. *Take the baby immediately to the emergency room.* Older children complaining of persistent joint or bone pain may also have an infection (septic joint or osteomyelitis). *Seek immediate medical help.*

Beyond the serious bone and muscle pains, parents also need to handle the everyday bruises, injuries and pulled muscles of childhood. Pediatric integrative pain expert Joy Weydert, M.D., recommends the following. *As always, however, check*

with your pediatrician before giving your child any herbs, supplements or homeopathic remedies.

Treating the Shock, Bruises and Pain of Injury

- *The homeopathic remedy arnica.* Use 30 C dose, 3 to 5 pellets orally every few hours initially, then four times a day until the child feels better. Homeopathic arnica ointments, containing arnica oil, are also available for use on the skin.
- *A warm bath with Epsom salts (magnesium salts).* This is absorbed through skin to relax muscles and relieve pain. Put 1 to 2 cups of Epsom salts in a tub of comfortably warm water for soaking.
- *Magnesium supplements (in the form of glycinate, gluconate, aspartate, oxide).* This is a natural muscle relaxant and pain reliever. The recommended dose is 250 to 500 milligrams orally, twice a day. (May cause diarrhea in some children.)
- *Bromelain enzyme.* This enzyme, found in pineapple, decreases pain, swelling and tenderness. It is available in prepared capsules taken orally. Follow package instructions for children.

- *Bach Rescue Remedy*. This flower essence eases stress and panic after trauma. Give 4 drops under the tongue.
- *Vitamin C and bioflavanoids*. In his useful book, *The Green Pharmacy*, botanist James A. Duke, Ph.D., recommends eating fruits that are rich in vitamin C and bioflavanoids in the treatment of bruises. "Together, these nutrients help strengthen capillary walls, making them more resistant to the blood leakage that causes bruises. When bruises occur, vitamin C and bioflavanoids help capillary walls—and black and blue marks— heal more rapidly."[43]

Easing Minor Pain and Inflammation of Muscle Spasms

- *Feverfew*. This herb relieves minor pain and muscle spasms. Give the extract or capsules three to four times a day orally, following package dosing instructions.
- *Turmeric*. Many clinical studies agree that the curcumin in turmeric has anti-inflammatory effects. But, as botanist James Duke, Ph.D., says, "It takes more than a shake of the spice

jar to gain this benefit."[44] For children, Dr. Weydert recommends 1/2 to 1 capsule one to three times daily taken orally.

- *Licorice tea*. Another way to relieve inflammation. Children can be given 1 cup twice daily orally for five to seven days only.
- *Herbal rubs can be used on the skin for muscle pain*. Dilute a few drops of the following essential oils in a tablespoon of vegetable oil:
  - *St. John's wort oil*. A pain reliever and anti-inflammatory, this oil is also good for growing pains and sleep problems.
  - *Arnica oil*. Use for bruises, muscle aches. This should only be used on unbroken skin.

Treating Wounds, Cuts, Scrapes, Burns

- Make sure the last *tetanus booster* was not given more than ten years ago.
- *Gaping wounds* or *wounds with a flap* need stitching. It is important to go to an emergency room immediately because the wound has to be closed within six hours.
- *Rinse* wound with clean, cold water; if necessary, remove debris with a clean soft brush.

- Use tea tree oil as a *disinfectant* (unless there is a known allergy, and not on children under age two).
- If the cut is still bleeding or oozing, cover with an *adhesive bandage* or sterile gauze. But it is preferable to let the wound dry and heal open to the light.
- *No sugar, white flour and dairy* during the healing time.
- *Burns:* Hold under running, cold water or in a basin with ice water until uncomfortable. This might have to be repeated frequently for several hours, every time the burn starts hurting again; over time, the periods of comfort will increase. If the burn is large (greater than two inches) or is on the face, genitals or palm of the hand, or if there are blisters, see a physician.

11

THE TOLL OF
STRESS ON CHILDREN:
"I CAN'T GO
TO SCHOOL TODAY"

In addition to all of the specific conditions discussed so far, parents are often faced with children who simply want to stay home and not go to school. Perhaps they are uncomfortable, or something hurts, or they have a problem like fibromyalgia, which causes pain and fatigue throughout the body. We know that stress— whether from home, school or other factors—contributes to chronic disease in children, but it is often hard to pinpoint the connection between stress and such conditions as digestive problems, headache pain or sleeplessness. My feeling is that no one knows your child better than you do, and this is a good time for you to trust your instincts, talk to your child, observe his or her behavior and demeanor at different times of the day, and—perhaps in consultation with your pediatrician—begin to unravel the complex relationships among your child's life experiences and his or her health. For example, do the symptoms go away when your child is on vacation or playing video games? When do they come back?

Dr. Joy Weydert, director of Integrative Pain Management at Children's Mercy Hospital, advises parents to focus on the level of functioning of the child. "How many of the activities at school or after school can the child participate in?" she asks. "For many of the children I treat, the level of functioning improves long before their level of pain decreases. Our bodies are wise and can do more than we think, but often, kids still need the pain complaint to keep getting the kind of attention they want. This is not a conscious thought for children, but we all need love and attention, and having a pain complaint often gives children that."

Dr. Weydert attributes many pain complaints of children to their reactions to the tremendous academic and social stress they face every day, at school and in the community. "When children are under stress for long periods of time, their sympathetic nervous systems go into 'overdrive,' pumping out stress hormones, causing tight muscles and digestive problems. This puts the body out of balance, as if it is constantly running a marathon. There is no opportunity to relax, recover and repair damaged cells. The body is taxed and the immune system is compromised. The result is aching muscles, sleep and appetite disturbances, upper respiratory infections, and digestive problems," says Dr. Weydert. "The body is not meant to take this kind of punishment."

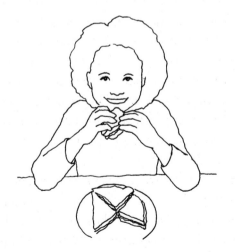

The solution seems intuitive: As a parent, do everything you can to create a peaceful, pleasant, nurturing home environment as a counterpoint to the stresses of your child's world outside the home. Calm family mealtimes—without television—and quiet places to do homework can help. Studies have shown, in fact, that kids in families that have sit-down dinners together are far less likely to smoke, drink and take drugs than kids whose families have more haphazard lifestyles. Regular family mealtimes also result in better grades and nutritional habits among children. If you are not convinced, here are ten benefits of family mealtimes supported by research at the Columbia University Center on Addiction and Substance Abuse.

Ten Benefits of Frequent Family Dinners

The more often children and teens eat dinner with their families, the less likely they are to smoke, drink and use drugs. Children and teens who have frequent family dinners:

- Are at half the risk for substance abuse compared to teens who dine with their families infrequently.

- Are less likely to have friends or classmates who use illicit drugs or abuse prescription drugs.
- Have lower levels of tension and stress at home.
- Are more likely to say that their parents are proud of them.
- Are more likely to say they can confide in their parents.
- Are likelier to get better grades in school.
- Are more likely to be emotionally content and have positive peer relationships.
- Have healthier eating habits.
- Are at lower risk for thoughts of suicide.
- Are less likely to try marijuana or have friends who use marijuana.[45]

Another way to create a peaceful, nurturing family environment is to help your child wind down in the evening and get a good sleep. (See Chapter 9, "I Can't Sleep," for suggestions of how to do this.)

12

FINDING AN INTEGRATIVE PEDIATRICIAN AND ALTERNATIVE PRACTITIONERS

If you like the perspective of this book, you might want to find an integrative (also called holistic) pediatrician. The approach of integrative medicine for children is to be concerned not only with the child's physical health, but also the health of the child's mind and spirit. In this chapter, I will give you some guidelines about what to look for and how to find someone in your area.

On his very useful Web site, Holistic Child Health (*www.holisticchildhealth.com*), Lawrence B. Palevsky, M.D., FAAP, president of the Holistic Pediatric Association, describes some of the reasons parents choose integrative pediatricians:

"The practice of medicine is changing and so is the relationship between parents and their children's medical health care practitioners. I want to acknowledge children have greatly benefited from the advancements of Western medicine through improvements in:

- The care of premature infants, sick newborns, and intensely ill children and teens
- The technology for better diagnostic procedures and cutting-edge treatments
- The development of lifesaving surgical procedures
- The treatment and understanding of genetic conditions
- The advancement of pharmaceuticals to treat children's complex conditions

"Increasing numbers of parents, caregivers and practitioners, however, are seeking answers to many child health care issues that go beyond the scope of Western medical practice. People want to be better informed about:

- The choices you can make about children's health care
- What you can do to help prevent and safely treat common childhood illnesses

- How you can help strengthen children's immune systems
- How your children get sick, get well and stay well
- How you can learn to safely address common and complex childhood illnesses
- What treatments are available for children in addition to Western medicine
- Why there is such an increase in chronic childhood illnesses
- What role nutrition plays in maintaining family health and treating illness
- How environmental factors affect children's health
- How the body/mind/spirit connection impacts family health
- How to get the doctor to listen, spend more time and respect differing opinions
- How to raise healthy children without the threat of debilitating conditions and the need for constant medications and therapies"

Dr. Palevsky's Web site also has very good descriptions of holistic medicine and the kind of relationship you can expect from an integrative/holistic pediatrician.

The problem that many people face is how to find integrative/holistic pediatricians in their home areas. The good news is that the number of doctors with an integrative orientation is growing, thanks to programs in integrative medicine such as Dr. Andrew Weil's in Arizona. So as a first step, I suggest that you look at this Web site that lists the graduates of Dr. Weil's program and where they are in the world: *www.integrativemedicine.arizona.edu/alum/index.html*. This list includes all specialties, not only pediatrics, but if you can find a graduate of this program in your area, perhaps he or she can recommend an integrative pediatrician.

For more guidance on finding an integrative pediatricians, I also suggest perusing the Web site of the Children's Hospitals and Clinics of Minnesota (*www.childrenshc.org/Communities/IntegrativeMed.asp.*), where you will find such useful information as a description of integrative pediatrics; a Children's Healing Helpline offering resource information and general questions about complementary therapies for children, (612) 813-7887 or 1 (888) 554-7887; and a list of publications written for young children and adolescents on a wide variety of complementary therapies.

You can also check the following Web sites for holistic practitioners specializing in children:

www.hpakids.org/index.html.

http://web.memberclicks.com/mc/directory/viewallmembers. do?masthead=true&hidOrgID=hpa

And finally, here are two additional Web sites that list other certified holistic practitioners, if you want to add alternative treatment providers to your integrative health care team:

www.holisticmedicine.org/ahma/public?action=findDoctors

www.holisticmed.com/www/directory.html

Parting Thoughts

The important thing to keep in mind in your search for health providers for your children is that you are a vital member of the team. The best health outcomes for children happen when parents see themselves as collaborators with their pediatricians, rather than as merely the recipients of instructions and advice. No one knows your children better than you do, so by working in partnership with your pediatrician, you can not only help your children become whole and healed, you can also teach your children how to take responsibility for their own health. You will be giving them a gift that will last a lifetime, the gift of "owning their health."

RESOURCES

Complementary and Alternative Medicine Web Sites

Academy for Guided Imagery *www.healthy.net/agi*

American Academy of Osteopathic Medicine
www.aacom.org/om.html

American Association of Naturopathic Physicians
www.naturopathic.org

American Botanical Council *www.herbalgram.org*

Berkeley Wellness Letter
www.wellnessletter.com/html/ds/dsSupplements.php

Columbia University
www.rosenthal.hs.columbia.edu/Botanicals.html

Consumer Labs (subscription)
www.consumerlab.com/index.asp

Council for Responsible Nutrition *www.crnusa.org*

Dr. Weil *www.drweil.com/u/Home*

Herb Research Foundation *www.herbs.org*

Herbal Materia Medica
www.healthy.net/clinic/therapy/herbal/herbic/herbs

Holistic Kids (Boston) *www.holistickids.org*

M. D. Anderson Cancer Center
   www.mdanderson.org/departments/cimer

McMaster University
   www-hsl.mcmaster.ca/tomflem/altmed.html

Memorial Sloan-Kettering Cancer Center
   www.mskcc.org/mskcc/html/11570.cfm

National Center for Complementary and Alternative
   Medicine (Herbal Supplements)
   www.nccam.nih.gov/health/supplement-safety

Natural Medicine Comprehensive Database (subscription)
   www.naturaldatabase.com

Office of Dietary Supplements *http://dietary-supplements.*
   info.nih.gov/Health_Information/IBIDS.aspx

Osteopathic Educational Services *www.osteohome.com*

University of Pittsburg *www.pitt.edu/~cbw/database.html*

Complementary and Alternative
Medicine Publications

Ditchek, Stuart H., and Russell H. Greenfield. *Healthy
   Child, Whole Child: Integrating the Best of Conventional
   and Alternative Medicine to Keep Your Kids Healthy.*
   New York: HarperCollins, 2002.

Freeman, L. W. *Best Practices in Complementary and
   Alternative Medicine: An Evidence-Based Approach with*

Nursing CE/CME. Gaithersburg, MD: Aspen Publications, 2001.

Freeman, L. W., and G. F. Lawlis. *Mosby's Complementary and Alternative Medicine: A Research-Based Approach.* St. Louis, MO: Mosby, 2001.

Jarmey, Chris, and John Tindall. *Acupressure for Common Ailments.* New York: Fireside, 1991.

Jonas, Wayne B., and Jeffrey S. Levin. *Essentials of Complementary and Alternative Medicine.* Baltimore, MD: Lippincott Williams & Wilkins, 1999.

Pelletier, Kenneth R. *The Best Alternative Medicine: What Works, What Does Not.* New York: Simon & Schuster, 2000.

Sumar, Sonia. *Yoga for the Special Child.* Buckingham, VA: Special Yoga Publications, 1998.

Weisman, Roanne, and Brian Berman. *Own Your Health: Choosing the Best from Alternative & Conventional Medicine.* Deerfield Beach, FL: HCI Books, 2003.

Worwood, Valerie Ann. *Aromatherapy for the Healthy Child.* Novato, CA: New World Library, 2000.

Baby Massage

Auckett, Amelia D., and Tiffany Field. *Baby Massage: Parent-Child Bonding Through Touch.* New York: Newmarket Press, 2004. You can also order Dr. Field's video, *Baby Massage and Exercise* (Activideo, 1989), via *Babies Today* and *Amazon.com.*

McClure, Vimala Schneider. *Infant Massage: A Handbook for Loving Parents*. New York: Bantam, 2000. A very popular book, recently expanded and updated, including fascinating new research about the effects of touch on parent/child bonding, infant stress, sensory development and the care of special-needs babies.

Walker, Peter. *Baby Massage: A Practical Guide to Massage and Movement for Babies and Infants*. New York: St. Martin's Press, 1996. This book details a simple, effective and safe way for parents to discover the magic and healing powers of gentle, loving touch. Twenty-one color photos and more than one hundred detailed line illustrations.

Walker, Peter, and Janet Balaskas. *The Book of Baby Massage: For a Happier, Healthier Child*. New York: Kensington Publishing, 1998. Cowritten by the founder of Britain's Active Birth Centre.

Guided Imagery, Biofeedback and Visualization

Curran, Ellen. *Guided Imagery for Healing Children and Teens*. Hillsboro, OR: Beyond Words Publishing, 2001.

Klein, Nancy. *Healing Images for Children: Teaching Relaxation and Guided Imagery to Children Facing Cancer and Other Serious Illnesses*. Watertown, WI: Inner Coaching, 2001.

Rossman, Martin L. *Guided Imagery for Self-Healing*. Tiburon, CA: H. J. Kramer, 2000.

Herbs

Duke, James A. *The Green Pharmacy*. Emmaus, PA: Rodale, 1997.

Garland, Sarah. *The Herb Garden*. New York: Penguin USA, 1996.

Levy, Juliette deBairacli. *Common Herbs for Natural Health*. Woodstock, NY: Ash Tree Publishing, 1997.

Levy, Juliette deBairacli. *Nature's Children*. New York: Warner Paperback Library, 1997.

McCaleb, Robert, Evelyn Leigh and Krista Morien. *The Encyclopedia of Popular Herbs*. Roseville, CA: Prima Health, 2000.

Murray, Michael T. *The Healing Power of Herbs: The Enlightened Person's Guide to the Wonders of Medicinal Plants*. Roseville, CA: Prima Publishing, 1995.

Robbers, James E., and Varro E. Tyler. *Herbs of Choice: The Therapeutic Use of Phytomedicinals*. Binghamton, NY: Haworth Press, 1996.

Twitchell, Paul. *Herbs: The Magic Healers: The Complete Guide to Physical and Spiritual Well-Being*. New York: Lancer Books, 1971.

Tyler, Varro E. *The Honest Herbal*. Binghamton, NY: Haworth Press, 1993.

Homeopathy

Jacobs, J., et al. "Treatment of Acute Childhood Diarrhea with Homeopathic Medicine: A Randomized Clinical

Trial in Nicaragua." *Pediatrics* 93 (1994): 719–725.

Jacobs, J., et al. "Homeopathic Treatment of Acute Childhood Diarrhea: Results from a Clinical Trial in Nepal. *The Journal of Alternative and Complementary Medicine* 6.2 (2000): 131–139.

Jacobs, J., D. Springer and D. Crothers. "Homeopathic Treatment of Acute Otitis Media in Children: A Preliminary Randomized Placebo-Controlled Trial." *Pediatric Infectious Disease Journal* 20.2 (2001): 177–183.

Jonas, Wayne B., and Jennifer Jacobs. *Healing with Homeopathy: The Doctor's Guide*. New York: Warner Books, 1998.

Linde, K., et al. "Are the Clinical Effects of Homeopathy Placebo Effects? A Meta-Analysis of Placebo-Controlled Trials." *Lancet* 350 (9081) (1997): 834–843.

NOTES

1. Data is from "Asthma and the Environment: A Strategy to Protect Children," President's Task Force on Environmental Health Risks and Safety Risks to Children, 1999.

2. A. H. Ernst, "Herbal Medicine for Asthma: A Systematic Review," *Thorax* 55 (2000): 925–929; and H. A. Cohen et al., "Blocking Effect of Vitamin C in Exercise-Induced Asthma," *Arch Pedtr Adolesc Med* 151 (1997): 367–370.

3. F. A. Paul et al., "Osteopathic Manipulative Treatment Applications for the Emergency Department Patient," *J Am Osteopath Assoc* 96 (1996): 403–409.

4. T. Field et al., "Children with Asthma Have Improved Pulmonary Functions after Massage Therapy," *J Pediatr* 132 (1998): 854–858.

5. K. A. Jobst, "Acupuncture in Asthma and Pulmonary Disease: An Analysis of Efficacy and Safety," *J Altern Complement Med* 2 (1996): 179–206.

6. T. Field et al., "Children with Asthma Have Improved Pulmonary Functions after Massage Therapy," *J Pediatr* 132 (1998): 854–858.

7. F. A. Paul et al., "Osteopathic Manipulative Treatment Applications for the Emergency Department Patient," *J Am Osteopath Assoc* 96 (1996): 403–409.

8. P. K. Vedanthan et al., "Clinical Study of Yoga Techniques in University Students with Asthma: A Controlled Study," *Allergy Asthma Proc* 19 (1998): 3–9.

9. K. A. Jobst, "Acupuncture in Asthma and Pulmonary Disease: An

Analysis of Efficacy and Safety," *J Altern Complement Med* 2 (1996): 179–206; and K. Linde, K. Jobst, and J. Panton, "Acupuncture for Chronic Asthma," *Cochrane Database Systematic Review* 2 (2000).

10. T. C. Ewer et al., "Improvement in Bronchial Hyper-Responsiveness in Patients with Moderate Asthma after Treatment with a Hypnotic Technique: A Randomized Controlled Trial," *BMJ* 293 (1986): 1129–1132.

11. Ibid.; and P. K. Vedanthan et al., "Clinical Study of Yoga Techniques in University Students with Asthma: A Controlled Study," *Allergy Asthma Proc* 19 (1998): 3–9.

12. M. I. Vazquez et al., "Psychological Treatment of Asthma: Effectiveness of a Self-Management Program with and without Relaxation Training," *J Asthma* 30 (1993): 171–183.

13. D. P. Kohen et al., "Applying Hypnosis in a Preschool Family Asthma Education Program: Uses of Storytelling, Imagery and Relaxation," *Am J Clin Hypnosis* 39 (1997): 169–181.

14. T. C. Ewer et al., "Improvement in Bronchial Hyper-Responsiveness in Patients with Moderate Asthma after Treatment with a Hypnotic Technique: A Randomized Controlled Trial," *BMJ* 293 (1986): 1129–1132.

15. B. Gintis, "AAO Case Study. Recurrent Otitis Media," *AAOJ* 6.2 (1996): 16.

16. V. Frymann et al., "Effect of Osteopathic Medical Management on Neurologic Development in Children," *J Am Osteopath Assoc* 92 (1992): 729–744.

17. L. M. Agresti, "Attention Deficit Disorder. The Hyperactive Child," *Osteopathic Annals* 14 (1989): 6–16.

18. R. W. Jarski et al., "The Effectiveness of Osteopathic Manipulative Treatment as Complementary Therapy Following Surgery: A Prospective, Match-Controlled Outcome Study," *Altern Ther Health Med* 6.5 (September 2000): 77–81.

19. G. P. Andersson et al., "A Comparison of Osteopathic Spinal Manipulation with Standard Care for Patients with Low Back Pain," *J Engl J Med* 341.19 (November 4, 1999): 1426–1431.

20. Edzard Ernst, ed., *The Desktop Guide to Complementary and Alternative Medicine: An Evidence-Based Approach* (Edinburgh: Harcourt Publishers Limited, 2001), 48.

21. Kenneth R. Pelletier, *The Best Alternative Medicine: What Works, What Does Not* (New York: Simon & Schuster, 2000), 198–199.

22. Ibid., 199–200.

23. Ibid., 201.

24. L. W. Freeman, *Best Practices in Complementary and Alternative Medicine: An Evidence-Based Approach with Nursing CE/CME* (Gaithersburg, MD: Aspen Publications 2001), Section 4-1, "Homeopathy—A Scientific Enigma."

25. Ibid.

26. Pelletier, *The Best Alternative Medicine*, 199.

27. J. Kleijnen, P. Knipschild and G. Rieter, "Clinical Trials of Homeopathy," *British Medical Journal* 302 (1991): 316–323. (Cited in Pelletier, *The Best Alternative Medicine*, 203).

28. Pelletier, *The Best Alternative Medicine*, 207–214.

29. Lixing Lao, "Traditional Chinese Medicine," in *Essentials of Complementary and Alternative Medicine*, Wayne B. Jonas and Jeffrey S. Levin, eds. (Baltimore and Philadelphia: Lippincott, Williams & Wilkins, 1999), 228.

30. K. J. Kemper et al., "On Pins and Needles? Pediatric Pain Patients' Experience with Acupuncture," *Pediatrics* 105 supplement (2000): 941–947.

31. A. C. Lee et al., "Survey of Acupuncturists: Practice Characteristics and Pediatric Care," *West J Med* 171 (1999): 153–157; D. Butkovic et al., "Comparison of Laser Acupuncture and Metoclopramide in PONV Prevention in Children," *Paediatr Anaesth*

15 (2005): 37–40; B. Duncan et al., "Parental Perceptions of the Therapeutic Effect from Osteopathic Manipulation or Acupuncture in Children with Spastic Cerebral Palsy," *Clin Pediatr (Phila)* 43 (2004): 349–353; K. J. Kemper et al., "On Pins and Needles? Pediatric Pain Patients' Experience with Acupuncture," *Pediatrics* 105 supplement (2000): 941–947; K. J. Kemperand and E. S. Highfield, "When Should You Consider Acupuncture for Your Patients?" *Contemp Pediatr* 19 (2002): 31–46; Y. C. Lin and B. Golianu, "Acupuncture as Complementary Treatment for Cyclic Vomiting Sydrome," *Medical Acupuncture* 13.3 (2002); D. Melchart et al., "Acupuncture for Recurrent Headaches: A Systemic Review of Randomized Controlled Trials," *Cephalalgia* 19 (1999): 779–786; D. K. Ng et al., "A Double-Blind, Randomized, Placebo-Controlled Trial of Acupuncture for the Treatment of Childhood Persistent Allergic Rhinitis," *Pediatrics* 114 (2004): 1242–1247; NIH Consensus Development Panel on Acupuncture, "Acupuncture Consensus Conference Report," *JAMA* 280 (1998): 1518–1524; S. Pintov et al., "Acupuncture and the Opioid System: Implications in the Management of Migraine," *Ped Neurology* 17 (1997): 129–133; A. Schlager et al., "Laser Stimulation of Acupuncture Point P6 Reduces Postoperative Vomiting in Children Undergoing Strabismus Surgery," *Br J Anesth* 81 (1998): 529–532; S. M. Wang et al., "Parental Auricular Acupuncture as an Adjunct for Parental Presence during Induction of Anesthesia," *Anesthesiology* 100 (2004): 1399–1404; and S. M. Wang and Z. N. Kain, "P6 Acupoint Injections Are as Effective as Droperidol in Controlling Early Postoperative Nausea and Vomiting in Children," *Anesth* 97 (2002): 359–366.

32. Sandra Blakeslee, "Complex and Hidden Brain in Gut Makes Stomachaches and Butterflies." *The New York Times*, 23 January 1996: 1.

33. Lynda W. Freeman, *Best Practices in Complementary and Alternative Medicine: An Evidence-Based Approach with Nursing CE/CME* (Gaithersburg, MD: Aspen Publishers, 2001), 3–1: 8.

34. Ibid.

35. K. Malkin, "Use of Massage in Clinical Practice," *British Journal of*

Nursing 3.6 (1994): 292–294. (Cited in Freeman, *Best Practices in Complementary and Alternative Medicine.*)

36. Freeman, *Best Practices in Complementary and Alternative Medicine,* 3–1: 8.

37. Ibid., 3–1: 7.

38. T. Field et al., "Massage of Preterm Newborns to Improve Growth and Development," *Pediatric Nursing* 13 (1987): 385–387. (Cited in Freeman, *Best Practices in Complementary and Alternative Medicine.*)

39. Edzard Ernst, ed., *The Desktop Guide to Complementary and Alternative Medicine: An Evidence-Based Approach* (Edinburgh: Harcourt Publishers Limited, 2001), 59–61.

40. A. Vickers et al., "Massage Therapy for Premature and/or Low Birth Weight Infants to Improve Weight Gain and/or Decrease Hospital Length of Stay," Cochrane Library (Oxford: Update Software, 1998). (Cited in Ernst, *The Desktop Guide.*)

41. T. Field et al., "Juvenile Rheumatoid Arthritis Benefits from Massage Therapy," *Journal of Pediatric Psychology* 22 (1997): 607–617.

42. M. Hernandez-Reif et al., "Migraine Headaches Are Reduced by Massage Therapy," *International Journal of Neuroscience* 96 (1998): 1–11.

43. James A. Duke, *The Green Pharmacy* (Emmaus, PA: Rodale, 1997), 98.

44. Ibid., 350.

45. Columbia University Center on Addiction and Substance Abuse*http://66.135.34.236/absolutenm/templates/PressReleases.asp? articleid=404&zoneid=56*

ABOUT THE AUTHORS

John D. Mark, M.D., is a Clinical Associate Professor of Pediatrics in the Pediatric Pulmonary Medicine division at Stanford University Medical Center. After completing his residency in pediatrics, Dr. Mark completed two fellowships; the first in pediatric pulmonology at University of Rochester School of Medicine and Dentistry and the second†in Pediatric Integrative Medicine at the University of Arizona program directed by Dr. Andrew Weil. Dr. Markís clinical and research interests focus on integrating alternative therapies and conventional therapies in the treatment of children with respiratory problems. In 2002, he was†awarded a grant from the National Center for Complementary and Alternative Medicine (NCCAM) for his project on guided imagery in children with asthma.

Roanne Weisman writes in the areas of science, medicine and health care. She is the principal author of the award-winning book, *Own Your Health: Choosing the Best from Alternative & Conventional Medicine* (HCI Books 2003). Her articles and feature stories have appeared in newspapers as well as in *Alternative Medicine Magazine, Body & Soul Magazine* and *Country Living Magazine*. She also writes extensively for the publications of most of the teaching hospitals of the Harvard Medical School. She has spoken and conducted workshops around the U.S. and in Canada on integrative medicine, which include her personal story of how "owning" her health helped her recover from a paralyzing stroke.